Counselling skills
FOR NURSES, MIDWIVES
AND HEALTH VISITORS

Counselling skills
FOR NURSES, MIDWIVES
AND HEALTH VISITORS

Dawn Freshwater

Open University Press
Maidenhead · Philadelphia

Open University Press
McGraw-Hill Education
McGraw-Hill House
Shoppenhangers Road
Maidenhead
Berkshire
England
SL6 2QL

email: enquiries@openup.co.uk
world wide web: www.openup.co.uk

and
325 Chestnut Street
Philadelphia, PA 19106, USA

First Published 2003

A catalogue record of this book is available from the British Library

ISBN 0 335 20781 2 (pb)   0 335 20782 0 (hb)

Library of Congress Cataloging-in-Publication Data
Freshwater, Dawn.
    Counselling skills for nurses, midwives, and health visitors / Dawn
    Freshwater.
      p. cm.
    Includes bibliographical references and index.
    ISBN 0-335-20782-0 (hbk.) – ISBN 0-335-20781-2 (pbk.)
    1. Nurse and patient. 2. Patients–Counseling of. 3. Midwives.
  4. Counseling. I. Title.

RT42.F658 2003
610.73'06'99–dc21

                                                        2002030417

Typeset by Graphicraft Limited, Hong Kong
Printed in Great Britain by Biddles Ltd, *www.biddles.co.uk*

This book is dedicated to all the patients with whom I have had the privilege of working.

Contents

Preface

Counselling has become part of the fabric of nursing.

(Burnard 1995: 261)

I was delighted to be asked by Michael Jacobs to write this book. Having trained to become a nurse over 20 years ago and being a practising counsellor for some 12 years I have often found it difficult to balance the boundaries between counselling and the use of counselling skills within the workplace. This is complicated by the fact that I have also been in academia for a number of years, supporting the development of undergraduate and postgraduate students in both an educative and pastoral role. Like many teachers and nurses engaged in education, I come across students experiencing personal difficulties, just as nurses, midwives and health visitors encounter patients in their everyday work whose life circumstances are causing a great deal of emotional, psychological, physical and sometimes spiritual distress. This book aims to outline the role that counselling skills can play in supporting, enabling and empowering patients and staff within the context of nursing.

When I refer to nursing, I use it as a broad term to incorporate a number of specialities; I also take the liberty of including health visitors and, for the sake of ease, midwives. The skills referred to throughout this text are transferable not only across disciplines but also within disciplines and, importantly, are just as helpful for supporting the practitioner as they are for the patient.

Having trained to be a counsellor over a decade ago, the biggest challenge and the aspect that I found most rewarding in the writing of this book was that of returning to the importance of creating an empathic relationship. While this is the most fundamental of all counselling skills, it is not easy to stay with what are often termed the more basic skills: a parallel that many nurses will recognize in relation to their own practice. As Winnicott, in his discussion of the analyst's knowing and not knowing notes

> When he [the analyst] has had several patients he begins to find it irksome to go as slowly as the patient is going, and he begins to make interpretations based not on material supplied on that particular day by the patient but on his own accumulated knowledge or his adherence for the time being to a particular group of ideas.
>
> (1965: 50–1)

Nursing too falls into this trap, approaching practice and the patient with a whole set of assumptions and paradigm examples from which to deduce the patient's needs. This text challenges the practitioner to put aside their assumptions and preconceptions and to go back to the foundations of nursing, that is, the nurse–patient relationship.

Egan, in *The Skilled Helper*, discriminates between the formal and the informal helper. Formal helpers are counsellors, psychologists, psychiatrists, social workers and members of the clergy. He notes that there are also informal helpers who 'deal with people in times of crisis and distress' (1994: 4). Here he includes doctors, dentists, teachers, police officers and importantly, for this book, nurses. He points out that 'Although these people are specialists in their own professions, there is still some expectation that they will help their clients or staff manage a variety of problem situations' (1994: 4). While this is a useful discrimination in relation to counselling, for the purpose of this book the various terms used to describe the carer (helper, practitioner, clinician and nurse) are used interchangeably. I would also like to point out that the clinical material that is used throughout this text in order to illustrate specific skills is based on fictitious patients and is based on my own experience of counselling within a healthcare setting.

I would like to thank various people who have offered their support and encouragement in the writing of this book. Thank you to Michael Jacobs, whose writing I found invaluable when in training as a counsellor, and whose editing has been support- ive and enabling. In addition, the friendship that both Michael and Moira Walker have extended to me over recent months has been very much appreciated.

Going back to my own training and early experiences of counselling, I wish to acknowledge Dilys Phipps for her insight and wisdom as a trainer and a colleague, and Sandra Griffiths and Vicki Gardiner. Thank you to Jeni Boyd who has been a sounding board for ideas, a proofreader, a colleague and a friend. Importantly, I would like to thank all those patients with whom I have had the opportunity to work over the last decade. I continue to learn and marvel at the mystery that is human relationship.

Dawn Freshwater

Chapter 1

Introduction

Communication is an essential part of healthcare, yet while it is recognized that good communication is fundamental to the caring relationship, in reality there are considerable variations in the quality of that communication and there is still the need for improvement. Skills derived from counselling are increasingly being used in nursing in an attempt to improve the level and degree of communication, and as such counselling skills are being taught in Project 2000 courses, bachelor's and master's degrees in health studies and post-registration continuing professional development (CPD) courses. Counselling skills have of course been used, perhaps in an unstructured manner, for many years in all branches of nursing including mental health, sick children's nursing and primary care as well as in health visiting and midwifery.

According to Buber (1958: 25), 'all real living is meeting'. The currency of this meeting is dialogue. Dialogue is not just about verbal and non-verbal interaction, but much more, as the physicist and cosmologist David Bohm (1990) notes in his work on wholeness and dialogue. Wholeness is not an unfamiliar concept in nursing; indeed many nursing practices, theories and philosophies are based on the principle of Holism. As I will demonstrate, many of the principles and concepts of counselling have influenced the development of nursing theory, nursing practice and nurse education.

This book explores aspects of counselling dialogue and how it might be used in a facilitative way within the context of healthcare, more specifically to facilitate holistic practice within nursing, midwifery and health visiting. While I refer to the fundamental philosophy of nursing, midwifery and health visiting as that of holism, this is not the place to debate the concept. Nevertheless the concept will be used to illustrate some of the ways in which counselling skills and the dialogic relationship might create the opportunity for authentic, congruent practice, something that many practitioners are experiencing as missing (Johns and Freshwater 1998) – witness the increasing problem of recruitment and retention within these professions. This book therefore, while focusing on the use of counselling skills for improving the patient's experience and the quality of care and of life, also attends to the potential of such skills for enhancing the meaning and satisfaction of caring for the practitioner.

A person's experience of herself or himself in this world is through psychological and physiological awareness, contained within a reflexive dialogue with both the self and the outside world. Cole (2001: 11) argues that:

> The presence of dialogue offers the *possibility* of balance, a state of equilibrium, a stress-less state. But the nature of the dialogue determines whether there is actually a balance, a state without stress, or whether a lack of balance indicates a state of stress.

The significant ⟨*In responding empathy?*⟩ urrent context is 'the nature of tl ⟨handwritten annotation⟩ on this aspect. If the nature of tl his is confirming and grounding for the patient. In responding empathetically, the practitioner stands alongside the patient, normalizing the struggle in which the patient is engaged, bringing the client back into the boundaries of being human.

Cook comments that 'many health professionals do not understand the value of counselling' (2001: 16). In order to work towards a better understanding of the use of counselling skills in nursing, midwifery and health visiting, this first chapter provides a brief overview of the status of counselling within these disciplines. While counselling skills form a substantial part of everyday practice for many health care practitioners, relatively few nurses are accredited counsellors. As such it is important to note that while this text refers to professional codes of conduct for counsellors and regulatory bodies, this book is not about the sort of counselling undertaken by professional counsellors. It is written for, and aims to support and supplement the skilled practitioner in the practice of their everyday work. For the novice practitioner it provides an insight into the counselling process, the therapeutic alliance and skills that may prove invaluable in the context of the nurse–patient midwife–family/mother and health visitor–client role. For the experienced practitioner it adds substance to the existing therapeutic expertise, while offering some contemporary reflections on the role of the counselling skills in nursing practice.

In October 1975 the Royal College of Nursing (RCN) set up a working party to:

> Explore further the concept of counselling within nursing with a view to providing information or producing recommendations for the attention of professional and official bodies which have the capacity to influence the development of counselling within the nursing profession.
>
> (RCN 1978: 7)

The report of the working party found that there were a number of misconceptions surrounding the use of counselling in nursing, complicated by the confusion regarding the term itself. They suggested that the term counselling, when used in ordinary conversation, denoted 'any interview or discussion which is undertaken to help people with problems' comparing this to the more restricted use of the term, which involves 'personal growth and development' (RCN 1978: 10). The confusion between counselling skills and counselling proper has existed and continues to exist in nursing as it does in other professions. The British Association for Counselling and Psychotherapy (BACP), in its earlier code of ethics for counsellors (1998) and for those using counselling skills in their functional role (1999), for example nurses, midwives and health visitors, has made clear distinctions between the two different uses of the term. More importantly BACP makes explicit the significance of the intention and aim behind the use of the counselling skills, which it argues is often to enhance the performance of the professional role of the practitioner rather than that of being a counsellor (BACP 1999). While many nurses use counselling skills as part of their daily work, acting as a counsellor is something very different.

Burnard (1995: 261) contends that:

> By the nature of their job, most nurses are involved in some form of counselling every day. A distinction has to be made, however, between exercising counselling skills and being a counsellor, and while nursing courses offer training in basic counselling skills, there is little or no training in how to be a counsellor.

Like the BACP, Burnard emphasizes the difference between the use of counselling skills and acting as a counsellor. Further, he indicates the significance of appropriate training, whether using such skills in a functional capacity to support a professional role or as a professional counsellor does. Nursing, midwifery and health visiting have their own professional code of conduct, which also identifies issues of patient safety, public protection and the extent and limits of any extension of the practitioners' role – something that the RCN working group (1978: 11) also raised, stating:

> When nurses counsel they require sufficient insight to recognise the extent and limits of their counselling skills, the dangers of exceeding those limits and knowledge of the availability of skilled counselling resources in their locality.

Thus there is the need for training, not only regarding the appropriate use of counselling skills in nursing, but also for the skills of being an effective reflective practitioner in order to be able to make discriminative assessments of clients' needs (and of their own capabilities). This is a critical component of the therapeutic relationship, as Bowman and Thompson (1998: 223) note:

> Generally, simple and appropriate information giving, teaching or counselling will have the greatest impact, but

knowing what is appropriate demands an understanding of the patient and their needs.

Nursing is about relationships, with both clients and colleagues; as such nurses need to develop self-awareness and interpersonal and emotional skills to cope with the sometimes difficult nature of their work. These skills can be developed within the context of reflective practice and clinical supervision, topics that are widely written about in the nursing literature and are central to the practice of counselling. As such they are referred to throughout this book.

Defining counselling

There are any number of descriptions of counselling, making it difficult to outline a simple definition. It is also worth noting that although there are numerous schools of psychological thought and frameworks within which counselling can take place, definitions of counselling are usually generic, covering a broad range of skills and theories. The British Association for Counselling and Psychotherapy provides a reasonably accessible definition of counselling:

> An interaction in which one person offers another person time, attention and respect, with the intention of helping that person explore, discover and clarify ways of living more successfully and towards greater well being.
>
> (Palmer *et al.* 1996: 22)

Other definitions of counselling focus on the therapeutic relationship, on what happens between the helper and the client (Jones 1970), while others take account of the underlying aims and values of counselling. Thus counselling can be described as a process which provides help and support, and an understanding listener for someone who is concerned, confused or perplexed. Creating a climate within which the individual can feel accepted, counselling helps clients to gain clearer insight into themselves and their situation, so that they are better able to draw on their own resources to help themselves. In this way counselling is contrasted with advice giving, opinion giving, sympathizing and giving practical help.

The role of counselling in nursing

Writing of the counselling role in nursing, Slevin (1995: 415) says:

> Here the nurse encourages the patient to examine his/her problems, conflicts or difficulties and to develop an awareness and understanding of these issues. Through addressing these problems, the patient is encouraged to work through them toward an awareness of the conditions essential to his/her health and wellbeing and how these conditions can be achieved.

Many nursing theorists have developed the notion of the therapeutic alliance, as identified within counselling, into frameworks for therapeutic nursing practice; this is particularly the case in mental health nursing. Peplau (1962, [1952]1988) is one such theorist, who, drawing upon psychodynamic psychology, outlines an interpersonal model of nursing based on professional closeness. Peplau views the therapeutic relationship as a highly structured situation in which the nurse adopts a professional stance. Subsequent nursing theorists have utilized humanistic psychology (see for example Paterson and Zderad 1988, Watson 1979 and Benner 1984) and behavioural models (for example Orem 1971 and Henderson 1966) in describing the nurse–patient interaction.

Studies examining the role of counselling in nursing and nurses' experiences of counselling suggest that counselling can 'assist individuals to *clarify* various aspects of their life-world', provide '*hope and encouragement*' and offer '*comfort*' or *support*' (Burnard 1998b; Soohbany 1999: 35, original emphasis). Several authors point out the similarities between nursing and counselling, noting that:

> Nursing, like counselling, is an interpersonal process that is aimed at assisting the individual in dealing with crisis and/

or coping with life traumas. It is also aimed, if necessary, at finding meaning in an experience. The aim of both is achievable through human-to-human relationships and this, in turn, is achieved through transcending roles of counsellor/ nurse and patient/client in order to establish caring presence and through making therapeutic use of self. Implicit in these relationships are the ability to listen, understand and respond as well as intervene purposefully.

(Soohbany 1999: 39; see also Soohbany 1996 and Jones 1993)

Creating and maintaining a climate within which the skills of counselling can be used effectively is an essential part of the interpersonal process, and is something that is attended to in more detail in subsequent chapters. Both directive and non-directive skills may be appropriate to use within nurse–patient encounters; both have a facilitative component. The non-directive personal development approach, which aims to empower, can be used to achieve optimal health in difficult circumstances such as chronic and terminal illness, disability and bereavement. This non-directive approach is largely derived from the work of American psychologist Carl Rogers ([1961]1991) and his person-centred approach that has formed the basis of humanistic nursing (Watson 1979; Paterson and Zderad 1988).

The emphasis of the non-directive approach is on the person and their natural capacity to come to terms with and solve their own problems. Thus the role of the nurse using non-directive counselling skills is that of acting as a catalyst and change agent for the client. A more directive approach to the use of counselling skills might be called upon for preventative health care in a wide range of nursing activities. The increasing use of cognitive-behavioural techniques (Beck 1976) in general has heralded the recruitment of a number of nurse therapists (again concentrated in the mental health field in the main) who are skilled in the use of directive approaches. The two approaches can of course be used to complement each other.

The counselling frameworks for understanding and exploring a client's experience are numerous but fall into three broad categories: psychodynamic, person-centred and cognitive behavioural (further reading around these theoretical orientations can be found in the final section of this book). Similarly, counselling skills can be crudely arranged into three groups: those of relationship building, exploring and clarifying, and action skills. These skills are examined in turn in later chapters, with specific emphasis on their application to nursing and the helping relationship.

While there are similarities between the disciplines of counselling and nursing, there are as many specialisms within nursing as there are theories of counselling. Hence it is worth exploring the various ways in which counselling skills may be reflected within the differing aspects of nursing work.

Counselling and health promotion

Much nursing work is concerned with health promotion, which in turn is about providing support and helping people to change behaviours that are detrimental to their health, such as smoking or drinking too much alcohol. Sidell reminds us that, 'There is a great deal of scope for using counselling skills to promote health in the everyday encounters health professionals have with their clients'. She goes on to provide examples, saying that, 'Community nurses may need to counsel someone who is having to deal with incontinence. Health visitors counsel on the immunisation of infants' (1997: 134). Another example is nurses engaged in family planning who use counselling skills to enable the client to make an informed decision about their sexual and reproductive health.

There is some evidence to suggest that clear and effective communication is of practical importance when both nurse and patient are faced with issues of *concordance* with treatment plans (Horder and Moore 1990). Hence counselling skills used in health promotion do not always originate from the person-centred philosophy as one might expect. Rather they draw upon both directive and non-directive skills, particularly as many health professionals are under pressure to achieve the Health of the Nation targets (DoH 1992). Those aimed at facilitating change, for example, may be more directive, specifically targeting harmful behaviour. One example of directive counselling in health promotion and illness prevention is that of alcohol counselling, in which the health professional gives specific advice on the changes necessary to reduce health limiting behaviour (Prochaska and DiClemente 1984). On the other hand a more non-directive use of counselling skills may be used in family planning services.

Counselling in primary care and mental health

Personal counselling for health has emerged within the context of mental health nursing, the focus being on biographical approaches, enabling the client to reflect on their circumstances and review their present dilemmas, often in light of past experiences. Developments in primary care have meant that some primary care trusts have been given responsibility for the provision of local specialist mental health services (DoH 2000). Concurrently the National Service Framework (NSF) for Mental Health (DoH 1999) has been released, with Standards 2 and 3 of the framework demanding that primary healthcare teams will, among other things, develop the skills and competencies to manage common mental health problems, while the NHS acute services are tasked with rolling out access to psychological therapies. Thus these two enormous areas of expertise are brought together by the government in order to tackle the very real problem of managing the mental health of the population.

The NSF for mental health (1999) notes that one-quarter of routine GP consultations are for people with a defined mental health problem. Approximately 90 per cent of mental health care is provided by the primary care team, some of the most common illnesses presented being eating disorders, depression (including postnatal depression) and anxiety related problems (including obsessive-compulsive disorders, phobia and panic related-symptoms). Patients have a number of access points in primary care, including the health visitor, district nurse, (increasingly) the practice nurse and the community psychiatric nurse (including the community mental health team). More and more professional counselling is also provided in primary health care (Bucknall 2001). Nevertheless the amount of patient referrals with mild to moderate mental health needs within primary care is also increasing, with nurses being the first point of contact for many of these individuals. A number of help lines have been set up as part of the increasing services, with nurses providing support through NHS Direct and NHS walk-in centres to patients and carers experiencing physical, emotional and psychological distress. It has been recognized that the requirement for basic and advanced training in counselling skills and cognitive behavioural therapy is critical to the successful implementation of these innovations, as is the need for adequate support and supervision of the staff working within these fields (DoH 1999).

Counselling skills and acute care

Nowadays counselling is a relatively commonplace part of hospital work. Although it is often those practitioners working within specialist areas such as cancer and palliative care, stoma care, gynaecology and neurology that have a specific counselling role assigned to their practice, there is scope for the use of counselling skills in almost every nurse–patient interaction, whatever the circumstances.

In 1990 Thompson's study indicated that a basic programme of in-hospital counselling undertaken by nurses working within a coronary care unit conferred significant benefits to both the client and their partner/relative. Similarly Cook (2001), a paediatric nurse also trained as a counsellor, reports on the inclusion of a nurse-counsellor in a paediatric intensive care unit. She draws on the work of Lansdown (1996), who specifies the ways in which using counselling skills with sick children and their relatives can provide families with much needed emotional and social support, particularly in the breaking of bad news.

Away from the high tech environment of intensive care, nurses and other health care professionals invariably find themselves engaged in teaching the patient and their families, whether this is about lifestyle changes following surgery or managing self-care routines. Teaching, however, is more than the transmission of information, and effective communication skills can go some way to ensuring that the patient is both able to retain and recall the necessary information. Counselling skills are not only an effective addition to these communication skills; they are also useful in monitoring the overall quality of the interaction between the nurse and patient. Thus educational counselling given by nurses improves knowledge and satisfaction (Raleigh and Odtohan 1987), reduces anxiety and depression for the patient and family (Thompson 1990) and can correct negative health habits (Carlssoin *et al.* 1997).

Midwifery and health visiting

Both midwives and health visitors encounter clinical situations every day, which demand a high level of interpersonal engagement. Midwives are finding themselves not only answering questions and providing support for parents having to make decisions regarding the health of their unborn child; they are also more often than not providing genetic counselling both antenatally and postnatally. On a day to day basis, the midwife is the first point of contact for the mother who is trying to make appropriate decisions about feeding and caring for her new infant. Health visitors support parents in their decisions surrounding immunizations, healthy development and schooling, not to mention postnatal family planning and general health. Of course, this does not take into account the many other aspects of these extremely diverse and challenging roles, but it does give an indication of the centrality of a good working relationship, and the skills required to maintain and sustain this.

This quick tour through some aspects of nursing work is by no means meant to be exhaustive. I am aware for example that a large part of the role of nurses, midwives and health visitors is dealing with loss and bereavement. It gives an indication nonetheless of some of the ways that counselling skills may enhance everyday nursing practice. The key concern of this book is to focus attention on the nurse–patient relationship and how the healing potential of this privileged position can be optimized through the utilization of 'intrinsic counselling' skills (Smith and Norton 1999: 18). The following chapters examine in some detail the counselling skills and processes that underpin the development of an effective therapeutic relationship. In Chapter 2 I discuss how to facilitate emotional solutions, usually reached by the patient through a non-directive approach, exploring how to help the patient find acceptable solutions to soluble problems and to learn to cope with insoluble ones. Successful counselling is a process that consists of stages and elements, which for the purposes of learning can be identified and separated conceptually. Chapter 2 examines some of the stages of counselling, linking them to theoretical models with the aim of outlining a framework for understanding the basic process. Concepts such as congruence, unconditional positive regard, transference and counter-transference are briefly considered, showing their relevance to nursing practice.

Establishing a rapport in the initial stages of a relationship requires the skills of active listening, good attention, and responding with genuineness and empathy. Chapter 3 concentrates on the counselling skills that may be used specifically in the early stages of forming a relationship, and then throughout the life of the therapeutic partnership. A significant part of any counselling intervention, whether the use of counselling skills in a professional role or as a professional counsellor, is the process of assessment in order that an appropriate decision can be made regarding the individual's treatment plan. Describing the skills of assessing through exploration and focusing, Chapter 3 provides practical examples of the skills of questioning, silence, summarizing, paraphrasing and reflecting that may be used in the establishment of basic empathy between nurse and patient.

Chapter 4 centres on helping the nurse to acquire the skills necessary to help patients piece together broad themes and relevant patterns and to develop new perspectives on their situation and on themselves. Skills such as self-disclosure, challenging, immediacy and pattern identification are addressed and linked to the notion of advanced empathy. Building on the development of alternative perspectives Chapter 5 explores the counselling skills required to facilitate action based on new understanding, including divergent thinking, decision-making processes and evaluation skills. The chapter also identifies the role of teaching, advising and information-giving within the nurse–patient interaction, including ways in which the practitioner may assist the patient to seek further support.

Over the last decade clinical supervision has been recognized and recommended as a central tenet of the continuing support and professional development of all nurses, midwives and health visitors (UKCC 1996). Chapter 6 attends to the function of clinical supervision within a practice that draws heavily upon counselling skills, emphasizing the professional issues that deserve to be considered within this context. Hence topics such as boundary concerns, ethical issues, confidentiality and record keeping, and the impact of future developments in nursing are debated.

This heralds the slight shift of focus to that of the concluding chapter, which is given over to the carer themselves. Caring for self is a significant concern for all professionals engaged in healthcare. This is even more so in the current climate of perpetual burnout and workaholism, leading to increasing anxiety regarding the recruitment and retention of staff. The RCN working party (1978) noted that nurses in training needed access to a counsellor and that staff counselling was in the main curative rather than preventative. Chapter 7 asks the question of the practitioner 'what do you do when you need to talk to someone?' Reference is made to the work of Isobel Menzies-Lyth (1988) regarding social systems as defences against anxiety; and to the Johari window in order to illustrate the importance of the development of self-awareness in nursing, with its potential of enabling the practitioner to cope with the interpersonal and emotional nature of work that is often difficult. Models of reflective practice are identified as one way of supporting the nurse in the development of their counselling skills, interpersonal communication and intrapersonal awareness.

Chapter 2

The process of counselling

As highlighted in Chapter 1, counselling is a process that consists of stages and elements that can help to guide and understand the development of a facilitating relationship. This chapter briefly outlines the stages of counselling, exploring the influence of theoretical models with the aim of identifying a framework for the basic process of counselling. This is then linked with relevant nursing theories and concepts, with illustrations from clinical practice. Many counselling skills and nursing skills are generic and can be taught and practised without emphasis on a particular theoretical model. They can also be applied and adapted to suit a diversity of contexts and settings. Nevertheless the inter-relationship between theory and practice is widely acknowledged, and in particular contemporary developments in nursing have been aimed at reducing the theory–practice gap (see for example Freshwater and Rolfe 2001; Rolfe *et al.* 2001).

The influence of reflective practice and clinical supervision on nursing is encouraging practitioners not only to develop intentional and conscious practice, but also to articulate their espoused theories and how they enact them. This clarification of values can be aided as the practitioner compares where their personal theories and those of others contrast and collide. This chapter, while not able to provide an in-depth examination of counselling theories, does aim to help the nurse to locate and clarify their view of the self and the self in relation to others.

Counselling models

In nursing numerous models have been developed by way of guiding the practitioner through the myriad of experiences that contribute to the nurse–patient encounter. Similarly a number of theoretical and philosophical models have been developed to inform the basis on which the processes and skills of counselling are derived. Models generally include a theoretical, a practical and a relational aspect (see Figure 2.1). A counselling model serves several functions. As well as acting as a structure for the counselling work and a framework for the use of skills, it can also act as a navigational aid for both the counsellor and the client as they work through the client's needs and purposes.

Nursing models also include a theoretical and philosophical component that underpins the practical and relational elements of the specified approach to nursing practice. Theoretical perspectives primarily represent attempts to define the practical aspects of day to day work. In counselling this is the counselling relationship, and the interface is between the actual experience

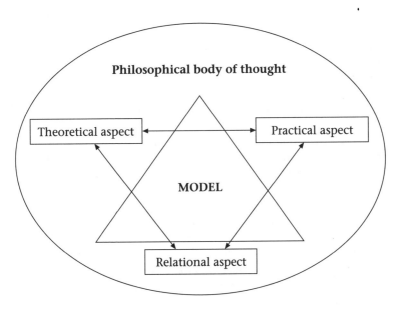

Figure 2.1 Components of a model

of a human relationship and the meaning that we make of that experience. This is of course similar in nursing, and it could be argued that nursing care has parallel aims, focuses and dynamics to counselling, despite its diversity of theoretical approaches. It is to some of these theoretical aspects that I shall now attend, drawing particular attention to some of the more obvious parallels between nursing theory and counselling theory so as to further locate the context of counselling skills within nursing.

What is a theory?

'Theory' is a generic term that is used to describe a notion or idea that explains experience, interprets observation and describes relationships. Traditionally a theory is an organized coherent set of concepts, which by their relationship to each other provide descriptions, explanations and predictions about phenomena. Thus theories are less abstract than models. They help us to understand and find meaning from our experience; they are a way of articulating our knowledge, and they stimulate questions that can lead to new insights (Parker 2001). Florence Nightingale taught that nursing theories explain and describe what is and what is not nursing (Nightingale 1859), while Parker contends that nursing theory 'describes and explains the phenomena of interest to nursing in a systematic way in order to provide understanding for use in nursing practice and research' (2001: 6).

Counselling theories inform the counsellor about concepts relating to human behaviour, about the principles of change and about basic assumptions surrounding the development of personality. However, any attempt at cognitive understanding is inevitably partial and as such no theory is 'the truth'; rather it opens up windows on to different 'truths'. In this sense it is important for the practitioner to assess and evaluate the usefulness of various theories against both their own experience and the current historical and social context. Further, it is important to realize the power that theory, and indeed the language used to describe theory has, to obfuscate and detract from experience. Theory provides a helpful map of the practicum, but should not be mistaken for the experience of practice itself.

There are three dominant approaches to counselling, each with theoretical, practical and relational aspects. They are the person-centred, the psychodynamic and the cognitive–behavioural approach.

Person-centred counselling

Theoretical aspect

Often referred to as Rogerian counselling after its founder Carl Rogers, the person-centred approach sits very much in the humanistic tradition. An influential psychologist and counsellor, Rogers became convinced during his career that human beings are essentially positive, forward-looking and realistic by nature. The fundamental premise upon which Carl Rogers based his theory was that the individual has within himself the resources for self-understanding, for challenging and altering self-concepts, attitudes and behaviours. This he called the actualizing tendency, which Rogers believed was the motivating force driving all human beings to achieve wholeness. Factors that inhibit or obscure the individual's actualizing tendency include the development of a negative self-concept. Accordingly person-centred counselling endeavours to help the client to become what they are capable of becoming, through releasing the psyche's own self-regulating mechanisms or 'the organismic self'.

Relationship to nursing

When viewed from a humanistic perspective, nursing can be seen as the ability to struggle with another through 'peak experiences related to health and suffering in which the participants in the nursing situation are and become in accordance with their human potential' (Paterson and Zderad 1976: 7). Nursing theorist Rosemary Parse captures this concept of 'potential' in her theory of 'health as human becoming' (1998). The goal of the nurse living out the theory of human becoming is 'true presence in bearing witness and being with others in their changing health patterns' (Parse 2001: 231).

Kleiman, an advocate of the humanistic approach to nursing, sees it as a call from humanity to maintain the humanness of the health care system, which she argues has become 'increasingly sophisticated in technology, increasingly concerned with cost containment, and increasingly less aware of and concerned with the patient as a human being' (2001: 167). So strong has the call to humanistic nursing been that the concept of a person-centred approach has been translated into patient-centred care in nursing (Pearson and McMahon 1998; Kirby 1999). But to truly realize patient-centred care means that nurses need to be working towards relationships that embrace the core conditions as outlined by Carl Rogers ([1961]1991) and summarized briefly below, and that acknowledge the client's own healing capacity. This means a significant shift from the medical model of cure to one of caring for the personhood of the client so as to support the development of their own healing potential (Freshwater 1998, 1999).

Another theorist who contributed significantly to both humanistic theories and person-centred counselling was Abraham Maslow. This is a very familiar name in nursing: Maslow's theory of motivation (1970) and hierarchy of needs (1968) are tools that most practitioners have used in some way in their everyday practice. The two concepts are often linked, the hierarchy of needs being related to motivation by two main forces: first, those that ensure survival by satisfying the basic physiological needs; and second, those that promote self-actualization or the realization of a person's full potential.

Maslow's hierarchy of needs (Figure 2.2) provides a useful framework for exploring the client's altering priorities through their experience of illness and disease. For example a patient who has undergone surgery is less likely to be concerned with peak experiences of self-actualization. Immediately postoperatively the client may be functioning at the level of physiological needs, where managing their pain and bodily functions becomes the main priority. Thus even though the patient may at some point have to face difficult issues around an altered body image, or the acceptance of a life-limiting illness, the timing of such a conversation is dependent on what specific needs are in the foreground for the client. Anyone who has experienced any sort of distracting pain, such as toothache or a headache, will

Need for Self-actualization Drive towards self-fulfilment Am I myself?
Recognition Needs The need to experience self-esteem and esteem of others Am I respected?
Belonging Needs The need to give and receive love Do I belong?
Safety Needs The need to feel secure and protected from harm Am I safe?
Physiological Needs Essential biological needs such as warmth, oxygen and food Will I survive?

Figure 2.2 Hierarchy of needs
(Source: adapted from Maslow 1968)

know that other higher level needs fade into the background until such time as the need to be free from pain is met.

When viewed within the context of mental health nursing Maslow's hierarchy takes on a different perspective. For some patients it is a struggle to remain conscious of their safety needs; indeed many of them are unable to maintain their own physiological needs, and so are admitted to acute psychiatric services for their own protection. Thus nurses may once again find themselves helping patients to maintain their basic needs, only in this instance for a different reason. This is particularly noticeable in the instances of patients with Alzheimer's disease and senile dementia.

The core conditions of person-centred counselling

The term empathy is employed variously in counselling, psychotherapy and across the helping professions. It is used to describe a particular characteristic that the helper should possess in relation to their client. In broad terms it is a state of being between two people, where one is entering the world of the other while maintaining an awareness of his or her own world. It entails the ability to see the world from the point of view of another individual, through their frame of reference, which in turn describes the ability of the helper to enter into the true feelings of the other person. It is not, however, an attempt to be that person, rather to enter an imaginative state 'as if' one were that person, and try to envisage how it might feel to be them. This notion of 'empathic resonance' is, according to some psychological theories, a basic and vital need 'in order to feel real, accepted and therefore valuable to others and in turn valuable to ourselves' (Jacoby 1984: 43).

It is the 'as if' quality that makes empathy different from sympathy. Sympathy, while concerned with feelings of pity, compassion and tenderness for the other person, often involves collusion, e.g. taking sides and becoming judgemental. Empathy requires 'much more effort, concentration and discipline' than sympathy and as such is not easy to accomplish (Hough 1994: 34).

It can be expressed or communicated through a number of key skills, some of which are outlined in detail in subsequent chapters. It includes active listening to both the words and the feelings that are being conveyed by the client. The reflecting back of the emotional content of the message from the client in the helper's own words enables the client to feel that their message has been understood. For the purpose of this book I split the practice of empathy into two parts, basic empathy and advanced empathy. Basic empathy is associated with the beginnings of a helping relationship and the building of trust. Advanced empathy is usually experienced once a relationship has been established and involves a considerable depth in understanding between the two individuals.

Given the transient nature of some relationships within nursing, it is likely that the majority of encounters within an acute hospital setting, especially in acute surgical settings, will be short-lived. While this permits only a brief interaction with the patient, it is still an ad hoc opportunity for the use of counselling skills. The nature of the nursing situation often encourages the early use of basic empathy. Patients are in vulnerable situations when in hospital, whether this is through an emergency or choice, as in an elective admission. It is very often the nurse who is best placed to spend time alleviating anxiety and caring for the emotional aspects of the individual's experience. Hence relationships, and relatively deep relationships, are formed swiftly, where empathic responses are an important feature. Longer-term caring relationships are formed with those patients suffering from chronic illness, both physical and mental, and indeed with families who have sometimes registered with the same primary health care team for decades. In these cases empathy is extended by more knowledge of a person's circumstances.

Advice and support is provided on an ongoing basis by, among others, the practice nurse, the district nurse, the school nurse and the health visitor who may develop deeply empathic relationships with patients who are part of their caseload.

Genuineness and congruence

No matter how skilled a practitioner may be in the use of counselling skills, empathic resonance is dependent upon the practitioner's warmth, genuineness and congruence. Sometimes referred to as genuineness, authenticity or transparency, congruence relates to the ability of the practitioner to be a real person in the helping situation. That is to say that the helper is not wedded to the idea of being the expert and does not assume a superior position in relation to the patient. In being honest with themselves, the practitioner is acting as a model for the patient, encouraging them to seek their own truth and to take risks in revealing hidden or painful aspects of the self (Rogers [1961]1991; Hough 1994; Sidell 1997). This is often difficult to achieve within the context of nursing, not least because the patient places the nurse in the position of expert, expecting them to know more about their care than they do. Of course the nurse does have access to information and knowledge that the client does not, which makes it difficult for them to respond to the client from a position of equality (Briant and Freshwater 1998).

There are also issues related to the power dynamics inherent within the nurse–patient relationship, just as there are in every helping relationship. I do not explore these particular dynamics in any great depth except in relation to professional boundaries, but further reading around this matter can be found in Guggenbahl-Craig (1978) and Jourard (1971).

Congruence is not always easy to achieve in everyday nursing practice, not least because nurses are often placed in positions where they have been asked to withhold specific information from a patient or relative, usually at the request of one or other of the family. When faced with direct questions from the people involved, it is hard for the nurse to remain congruent while simultaneously meeting the needs of the person he or she is caring for.

Unconditional positive regard

Unconditional positive regard, often described as acceptance, involves taking a non-judgemental stance towards the client, accepting them for who and what they are. Rogers ([1961]1991) believed that all of us have a right to be accepted for who we are and that this sort of prizing of the client is necessary for them to feel safe within any relationship. The key to achieving unconditional positive regard is linked to the ability of the helper to differentiate between the person's behaviour and the person themselves. Thus within the person-centred approach to counselling

> the client's behaviour may be viewed as something quite separate from or even alien to him, since behaviour is, in any case, contingent upon the current circumstances or difficulties which the person is experiencing.
>
> (Hough 1994: 34)

Nurses work with a diverse range of people from a wide range of social backgrounds and with differing beliefs and value systems around health, related for example to sexual behaviour or smoking and consumption of alcohol. Many patients continue with risky health behaviours despite having information about the negative and potentially damaging aspects of their actions. This may make it difficult for the nurse engaged in health promotion activities to continue to prize the patient. Indeed, it is possible that the patients' and the carers' beliefs and values may conflict altogether. One example might be the nurse who due to her strong Catholic faith finds it hard to practice non-judgementality in a gynaecological setting where patients are choosing to terminate their pregnancies. A further example is in the families who because of their faith in the Mormon religion choose not to accept some forms of treatment, despite the risk to life that this decision poses. In such complex situations working with a non-judgemental approach can prove problematic.

Practical and relational aspects

Humanistic approaches share a set of assumptions about human beings, which influence and shape the goals and style of the therapeutic relationship. Creating an atmosphere of safety through the use of the core conditions is a fundamental aspect of the helping relationship so as to enable the expression of feelings. Practising with a non-judgemental manner can facilitate the client to expand their awareness of themselves and develop an internally focused locus of control. As clients themselves become more congruent they also become more open, realistic, confident, and self-directing.

Many nursing practices are based on a similar relational model, drawing upon the work of Dorothea Orem (1971). Orem's self-care model is based on the belief that persons are expected to strive to retain self-resilience and as such nursing interventions may act for/do for another; educate, support or guide another and provide a developmental environment for another. The core conditions as expressed in the humanistic approach to counselling can help support the development of the caring relationship and the range of interventions, including compensatory nursing actions, while maintaining a stance of self-directed and patient-centred care.

Psychodynamic counselling

Theoretical aspects

Psychodynamic approaches were pioneered by Sigmund Freud, whose method of psychoanalysis is seen as the starting point for

The Conscious	Contains ideas and feelings in awareness at any particular time.
The Preconscious	Contains acceptable ideas, feelings and experiences which can become conscious through the process of reflection.
The Unconscious	Contains unacceptable ideas and feelings, experiences and repressed needs which may be recalled under certain therapeutic conditions.

Figure 2.3 Freud's topographical model of the psyche (1915)

all future work developed in the field of psychotherapy. Freud's theories and concepts have been modified and adapted over the years by a large number of theorists including Carl Jung, Melanie Klein, John Bowlby and Donald Winnicott. McLeod (1993) identifies three distinctive features of the psychodynamic approach. These are: that the client's difficulties have their ultimate origins in childhood experiences; that the client may not have a conscious awareness of their true motives or impulses behind their behaviour; and that the use of dream analysis, interpretation and transference in counselling may help the client to become more conscious.

The notion of conscious and unconscious processes were born out of Freud's (1915) early topographical model in an attempt to understand the mind. He later developed this model to include a structural model (1923). The main tenets of these models can be seen in Figures 2.3 and 2.4.

In brief, the ego experiences anxiety when it feels under threat from a perceived danger. Freud believed that the unconscious impulses and wishes of individuals can be defended against, and that defences are to cope with anxiety. As mentioned in Chapter 1, anxiety is one of the main reasons for individuals presenting themselves at their general practitioners (the other is

The Id	Contains inherited drives and is governed by the pleasure principle.
The Ego	Maintains the psychic balance between the demands of the Id, the Superego and external reality. Governed by the reality principle.
The Superego	Attempts to inhibit the Id and influence the Ego by setting moralistic values internalized from parental, cultural and social influences.

Figure 2.4 Freud's structural model of the psyche (1923)

depression). It is often when defences cease to function effectively that a person seeks help; in the patients presenting in general practice, this is sometimes because anxiety and other feelings are expressed through physical symptoms.

Denial is one such defence, frequently employed in order to avoid facing a distressing situation, causing thoughts, feelings and perceptions to be distorted. Examples of this include people who are dealing with their anxiety by obliterating it with intoxicants such as alcohol or drugs and who eventually suffer physical deterioration as a result.

> Kate, a 29-year-old mother, recently lost her second child during the final stages of labour. Desperate to get back to normal and to continue with the routine of taking care of Daniel, her 2-year-old son, Kate determined to 'get on with it' after the burial of her dead daughter. Despite repeated attempts by the health visitor and midwife to offer support to Kate and her husband, Kate insisted that she was coping well. Over time Kate's husband Dave became increasingly concerned about her mood and her difficulty in sleeping at night. He was particularly concerned about the amount of alcohol she was consuming to

'help her get to sleep', but was unable to persuade her to seek help. Unable to face food in the morning on waking, Kate soon got into the habit of not eating for long periods of time, finding that when she did eat she experienced some abdominal discomfort and acid regurgitation. Kate eventually presented to her doctor with what she thought was a stomach ulcer, which she said was waking her up in the night.

Rationalization is another example of how the individual can find reasons to justify their behaviour.

Stan, a 49-year-old man with circulatory deficits brought about by smoking, had recently undergone a below-knee amputation of his right leg following severe necrotic changes in his feet. Despite being advised to stop smoking, Stan continued to believe that his circulatory problem was caused by an accident he had when he was younger. He told himself that he needed to smoke because he had asthma, and when he had tried to give up in the past, he had found that this had exacerbated his asthma as he developed a cough. He was provided with evidence that a cough is a symptom that the lungs are repairing the damage done to them following years of smoking, but he chose to deny the evidence, stating that smoking helped him to breathe more easily.

Transference and counter-transference

Transference occurs in counselling when the client responds to the counsellor as if they were a significant person from the client's past. These feelings are likely to be present in any situation but are often evoked or exaggerated in cases where the client is vulnerable, for example in the experience of physical illness, mental distress or hospitalization (Rolfe *et al.* 2001). Counter-transference refers to feelings, behaviours and attitudes of the counsellor to the client. These responses may result from unresolved conflicts in the therapist's own life. Originally viewed as an impediment to the therapeutic relationship, it has recently been seen as a valuable indicator of what is happening between the client and the counsellor.

Relationship to nursing

Hildegard Peplau was an outstanding leader and pioneer in psychiatric nursing, whose career spanned many decades and whose model of therapeutic practice was developed with a group of women experiencing depression. Peplau ([1952]1988) focused on psychodynamic theories, viewing anxiety as a crucial influence in health and illness; positive anxiety is linked to healthy mental energy and productivity, and negative anxiety is associated with symptoms such as headaches, depression and insomnia. Kirby (1999: 413) suggests that

> The model presents the nursing response to this situation as one which involves the nurse–patient relationship as a vehicle for assisting the client toward resolution of this dilemma. That is, toward the unbounding of anxiety and the achievement of personal growth.

It is fair to assume that for many individuals the experience of ill health brings about a regression, that is to say the person goes back to an earlier state of emotional development; not least because the individual is suddenly forced into a position of dependency and reliance upon others. It is not surprising then that many clinical situations evoke transference and counter-transference responses in the patient together with the opportunity for the carer to assist the patient in managing themselves and their relationships differently. This potential was the subject of a paper in which Sayce (1993) argued that workers in mental health settings were in a unique position to help women who were sexually abused as children regain their confidence and self-esteem. Citing a study that identified that one in two women who sought help from the mental health services remembered being sexually abused in childhood, he argued that nurses should have access to opportunities for training and supervision to explore professional and personal responses to sexual abuse (Palmer *et al.* 1992).

Practical and relational aspects

The therapeutic relationship is characterized by the anonymity and the objectivity of the counsellor so that the client can project feelings and experiences on to them. The focus is on working through defences and the interpretation of transference and counter-transference as a means of understanding the client and enabling the client to expand their view of themselves. In this way the client is moved towards developing insight into their motives and patterns, and into reasons behind symptoms, emotions and impulses. Links are established between the past and the present and between the external and internal world of the patient.

In practical terms an understanding of the parallel processes between client–counsellor, client and significant others (past and present) can be obtained by analysing the interaction between transferential and counter-transferential responses (detailed explanations of these phenomena can be found in other texts: see for example Casement 1985; Jacobs 1991). Peplau ([1952]1988) viewed the therapeutic situation as a highly structured one and coined the term 'professional closeness' to describe a professional working relationship which is also based on intimacy and closeness. This may be one reason why practitioners often find the psychodynamic way of working uncomfortable, as the focus is on self-awareness and the therapeutic use of self. This can be quite demanding in that the practitioner needs to know and understand themselves in relation to others, including their counter-transferential responses and their own uncaring aspects (Rolfe *et al.* 2001).

Cognitive–behavioural counselling

Theoretical aspects

At the centre of cognitive–behavioural therapy is the premise that our interpretations of experience are hypotheses rather than facts, and therefore may be incorrect or correct to varying degrees. The assumption then is that the individual's view of the self and the personal world is central to their behaviour. Thus it is argued that the individual's problems are caused not by the situations themselves, but by the way in which they *think* about those situations. Albert Ellis (1990) called this 'distorted thinking'; Aaron Beck (1976) similarly described 'automatic thoughts'; whereas George Kelly (1995) operationalized his ideas through a theory of personal constructs, identifying the role of beliefs in behavioural patterns.

Cognitive–behavioural counselling has been linked to a problem-solving approach which Carkhuff (1987) developed and which Egan (1994) amplified, incorporating three stages to counselling, namely the present scenario, the preferred scenario and how to get there. This pragmatic model of helping provides a useful framework for the practitioner to hang their counselling skills on, always remembering that the interaction between the counselling skills and practitioner qualities is of utmost importance in the creation of a therapeutic alliance.

Relationship to nursing

Cognitive–behavioural therapy has recently become a central feature of everyday nursing practice, not least in the mental health field, where the NSF for Mental Health (DoH 1999) and the NHS Plan (DoH 2000) have set out clear expectations regarding the use of short-term psychological therapies to manage the increasing number of clients presenting with mild to moderate mental health problems. Childs-Clarke (1994) describes how he developed a cognitive–behavioural approach to the nursing care of patients with bulimia, stating that nurses 'are ideally placed to identify and respond to these problems' which are 'increasingly being encountered in clinical practice' (1994: 40). Cognitive–behavioural approaches can also be employed in a wide range of everyday nursing activities, especially in conjunction with learning theories that focus on conditioning and positive and negative reinforcement.

A practice nurse working within a GP's surgery might employ cognitive–behavioural skills to encourage a patient with a leg ulcer to embrace their treatment plan. Very often the dressing and cleaning of leg ulcers is a painful and uncomfortable procedure with often noxious smells adding to the unpleasantness of the experience. The practice nurse can reinforce the benefits of attending the clinic to the patient, emphasizing the positive behaviours and making the trip to the clinic a meaningful social interaction which aims to restore the patient's self-esteem as well as attend to their physical needs.

Practice and relational aspects

The aim of cognitive–behavioural counselling is to change the way the client thinks, with the counsellor striving to engage the client's active participation in all aspects of the work. Clients must be willing to experiment with new behaviours with counsellors who employ such action-oriented techniques as role-play, assertive and life skills training, modelling, homework assignments and positive and negative reinforcement. Many cognitive–behavioural theories do not hold that a warm relationship between the client and the counsellor is a necessary prerequisite to stimulate changes in thinking or behaviour, although in practice there is generally an understanding that an atmosphere of close collaboration and unconditional positive regard is desirable. This is a significant factor in the application of cognitive–behavioural skills to nursing situations, where the client is working to accept physical changes that are often aesthetically challenging.

Developing a framework for counselling skills

The skills that feature most obviously within the three main theories of counselling can be used interchangeably to complement each other at varying stages of the development of the therapeutic relationship (Figure 2.5).

Relationship building

At the beginning of a relationship the helper aims to establish a rapport with the client in order to build a connection that is based on trust and equality. This is achieved not only through empathic resonance, genuineness and unconditional positive regard, but by providing good attention (the practitioner needs to have cleared a physical and a psychological space so as to be

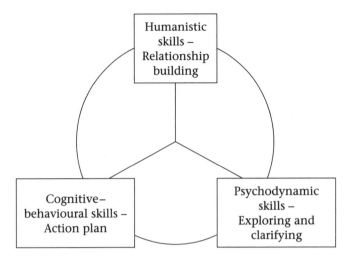

Figure 2.5 Stages of development in the therapeutic relationship

present to the client) and active listening. The establishment of a facilitative relationship is a basic requirement if other counselling skills are to be effective. This stage is 'non-directive and geared to eliciting the maximum amount of personal strength and confidence from the client' (Hough 1994: 40). These skills are described in more detail in Chapter 3.

Exploring and clarifying

As the relationship develops, the helper assists the client in piecing together an emerging picture, often bringing in broader issues or challenging the client when displaying contradictions or erroneous assumptions. The practitioner may also identify and confront the client with patterns that are beginning to emerge in the work. Chapter 4 addresses the skills of exploring and clarifying in depth.

Action skills

Based on a new understanding of themselves, the practitioner helps the client to act differently. Using a variety of skills to assist the client to set and achieve goals, the practitioner can guide the client in finding a way to work out a specific action strategy and ways of evaluating this. Skills used in earlier phases of the work are used in conjunction with decision-making and problem-solving skills, to enable the client to mobilize their own resources. These skills are explained further in Chapter 5.

Summary

Nurses, doctors, psychiatrists, mental health nurses and other health professionals do a great deal of counselling, in its broadest sense. The use of basic counselling skills, in conjunction with a sound theoretical understanding, can assist the nurse in gaining an awareness of the person as well as the problem; in promoting the ability to communicate and empathize with people from a variety of diverse backgrounds; and in recognizing patient's anxieties, including the anxieties they are almost bound to have regarding their health. Frameworks for guiding the practitioner in the use of their skills can provide a set of pathways for the nurse–patient interaction, as well as a means of assessing the effectiveness of the therapeutic relationship.

Chapter 3

Beginning a relationship

> The places where we are genuinely met and heard have great
> importance to us. Being in them may remind us of our strength and
> our value in ways that many other places we pass through do not.
>
> (Remen 1996: 242)

Establishing a rapport in the initial stages of a caring relationship requires, amongst other things, the skills of active listening, good attention, responding with genuineness and empathy. This chapter concentrates on the counselling skills that may be used specifically in the early stages of forming a relationship, and more generally throughout the life of a therapeutic relationship. A significant part of any counselling intervention, whether it is the use of counselling skills in a professional role or as a professional counsellor, is the process of assessment. This chapter therefore provides practical examples of the skills of questioning, silence, summarizing, paraphrasing and reflecting, and how they may be used in the communication of basic empathy between nurse and patient in the early assessment of the patient's needs.

Communication is what links us with other people and helps us to stay connected to society as a whole. There are many forms of communication and not all of them are speech related. There is a range of non-verbal communication skills which can be used effectively to get a message across without the use of language. Where language is used it can either serve to make people feel included or excluded. I begin by exploring accurate listening, perhaps one of the most important skills in establishing an inclusive relationship with another person, and one which consists of both verbal and non-verbal aspects.

Accurate listening

Listening is widely recognized as one of the basic abilities of anyone who claims to be interpersonally skilled (Burnard 1998a). Van Ooijen and Charnock (1994) suggest that there are three phases to therapeutic listening: receiving and understanding; communication of that understanding; and awareness in the other person that they have been heard and understood. Macleod Clark *et al.* (1992) further describe the levels of listening, as listening for facts, for feelings and for intentions. In *Swift to Hear*, Jacobs (1999) provides guidelines for listening which are useful in raising awareness of what *not* to do when attempting to establish a bond. The skills of active and accurate listening thus include:

• reflecting meaning;
• reflecting feeling;
• silence;
• questioning;
• paraphrasing;
• summarizing;
• ability to listen to oneself.

Using these skills enables the patient to hear their thoughts and feelings aloud in the context of an empathic situation. Active listening is however not just about hearing the words of the speaker; it is also about observing the use of body language, both the patient's and one's own.

Appropriate use of eye contact, for example, can be used to communicate to the patient that you are willing to engage with them. According to Hargie *et al.* (1986) this is the initial step in commencing an interpersonal interaction. Voice tone, pace and pitch can also do much to change the atmosphere of a situation. Nurses can also indicate with their body language that they are attending, for example by nodding, by facing the patient, by leaning forward and by using an open body posture. On the other hand raised eyebrows, insufficient eye contact or exclamations of surprise or shock can give negative feedback to the patient.

Hargie *et al.* (1986) describe a receptive atmosphere as one in which communication is enhanced and distractions are kept to a minimum. Distractions to active accurate listening can be both internal (within the nurse, physical, emotional and psychological) and external (the setting, noises, other pressing priorities). These are addressed in more detail in Chapters 6 and 7 in regard to self-awareness. Here I include a brief synopsis of counselling skills that might be used to create a receptive atmosphere.

Reflecting meaning

Reflecting back what the person has said is widely used as a counselling skill. Reflecting meaning communicates as briefly as possible that the listener has understood the key message being communicated by the patient. This can take the form of a question, or of selective 'echoing', and can be used to highlight what the nurse considers to be crucial words or points. For example, a patient is being prepared for discharge following surgery and says, 'I know my wound is healed, but it's still sore and red. What if something happens to it once I get home?' The nurse might respond, 'If something happens to it?' in the form of a question, encouraging the patient to be more explicit about their fears and anxieties. 'Yes, I am not worried about a bit of bleeding . . . that doesn't bother me. But now the stitches are out I am frightened it will pop'. This selective echoing allows the patient to expand upon their earlier question, outlining their fear of the wound bursting once they are discharged. The nurse is then able to offer information and reassurance directly related to the patient's meaning, rather than the nurse's assumption of what the question means.

Reflecting feeling

The purpose of reflecting feelings is to focus the patient's attention on the feeling rather than on the content alone, since it can help to raise awareness of vague unexpressed feelings that are not easy for the patient to acknowledge. In the following example, Paul considers that his diagnosis of HIV positive is to be expected. 'After all I am gay'. Even though he has remained faithful to his partner of the last 10 years, he says that it is well-known that gay men are more at risk of developing the disease. This is a rather rational response and the nurse wants to help Paul express his feelings concerning the diagnosis. So she may respond by saying, 'You feel because you are gay that you deserve to be HIV positive; you're almost resigned to it?' The nurse may be aware of other feelings that are around but not being expressed, perhaps about Paul's relationship, but she holds on to that awareness until such time as it seems appropriate to reflect on this with him.

Reflecting feeling back to a patient often elicits cathartic expressions of pent-up feelings and emotions, particularly in situations where distress has been contained for some time, for example in the case of the loss of a sick relative. As such the skill of simple reflection, when used in the context of a therapeutic relationship, has the potential to be a powerful facilitative intervention (Heron 1989). The release or outpouring that follows may surprise even the most experienced counsellor. Here it is perhaps pertinent to provide a brief overview of the significance of self-awareness and of knowing self when undertaking a counselling role.

Listening to self

Burnard exhorts the practitioner to 'stay awake' while listening. He goes on to say that 'it is vital that people *notice* their own feelings and thoughts, their own body position, posture, eye contact and so forth' (1992: 98). Staying awake in this way means that the nurse is more observant and attuned both to the needs of others and to their own needs. This developing sense of self-awareness may at first lead to the experience of self-consciousness. Learning new skills, or making previously taken for granted skills more conscious, invariably creates a degree of self-consciousness, causing some embarrassment and shyness. This self-consciousness however gradually develops into a continual process of noticing and examining aspects of the self with the purpose of deepening personal and interpersonal understanding.

Self-awareness as a topic has been widely written about in nursing and has gained momentum over recent years alongside the increasing awareness of reflective practice and the drive towards clinical supervision (Burnard 1992; Freshwater 2000; Heath and Freshwater 2000); see also Chapter 6, this volume. French (1983) asserts that awareness of the self enables the nurse to do three things:

- to make decisions on the most appropriate responses;
- to assess their personal abilities, limitations and training requirements;
- to obtain feedback on personal performance during skilled action.

Other writers take this discussion further, commenting on the value of the process of self-awareness in nursing for all parties concerned (Stewart 1983; Freshwater 1999, 2002). The process of raising self-awareness happens both through introspective means and with feedback from other people. Introspective acts of exploring one's own conscious processes reveal a whole range of mental experiences that are available for reflection, including thoughts, emotions, memories, images, problems, needs, wishes and desires. According to psychodynamic theory there is also a large amount of unconscious activity which, with some effort, can be recalled. Both conscious and unconscious material is an aid to self-understanding.

If we are to know ourselves, however, then we must also study ourselves in relation to other people. As Stewart points out, if nurses do not seek self-knowledge 'many of the patient's needs will go unmet because they are not recognised'. He goes on to say that 'perhaps needs go unrecognised when the nurse is unable to get to grips with some part of herself' (1983: 25) thus emphasizing the value of the introspective process.

Silence

Silence, which is a rarity in human interaction, particularly within busy health care settings, is a skill that provides a completely different experience for the patient. Silence can be a resting place for patients, a time when reflection can take place – but it can also be difficult to tolerate. While silence may encourage a patient to talk, it might also incite the practitioner to interject and fill what can feel like an uncomfortable empty space. Broadly speaking, silences can be separated into the following categories:

- passive;
- active;
- creative;
- destructive.

Positive silences, characterized by intimacy and harmony, feel comfortable and they encourage the patient and the nurse to become more aware of their inner worlds and of each other. In this sense the silence is active *and* creative. Negative silences are less comfortable and are associated with a tension that suggests animosity or hostility. The nature of a silence can be checked through a simple question. A simple 'What's happening?' or 'What are you feeling at this moment?' offers the patient the opportunity to say as much or as little about the silence as they feel able to. Alternatively the nurse might ask: 'Are you finding it difficult to put something into words?'

For example, Andrew, who has recently suffered a severe heart attack, is struggling to come to terms with the fact that he might not be able to return to his job as a train driver. He has asked to speak to his primary nurse, yet when they have some time together he is unsure of what to say. In the early stages of the relationship, the nurse might be aware that Andrew is afraid of getting in touch with his deep-seated fears and emotions concerning his future, and indeed with his mortality. At this early stage, however, it is important for the nurse to allow Andrew to go at his own pace, focusing on building a safe space for him to explore his fears and emotions. So when Andrew says that he doesn't know where to start, and remains silent for a minute or two, the nurse can respond by reflecting back to him, 'It's difficult for you to know where to begin'. This lets Andrew know that she is with him and prepared to wait for him to find a place to begin.

Open-ended prompts

Prompts to encourage the patient to continue speaking may include non-verbal encouragement such as nodding, or through echoing the last word or phrase said by the patient. Other prompts include 'yes', 'go on', 'and then . . .' Silence can also be used as a prompt, encouraging the patient to continue their train of thought without interruption. For example, Sarah is trying to decide whether or not to have her daughter immunized against measles, mumps and rubella. Her daughter has already had her initial immunizations and was well following them, but Sarah is concerned about the information that has to come light in recent media coverage, and she says to the health visitor: 'I think I just need to talk it through and get some reassurance; it's hard to keep focused on the real facts'. The health visitor might respond with a simple 'yes . . .' by way of encouraging Sarah to do what she says she wants, that is to talk it through. Sarah responds to the health visitor's prompt by saying: 'Well I thought I had it all straight in my head. I was fine when she had her first lots of jabs – no problem'. Sarah stays silent for a while. The health visitor allows sufficient time for reflection and then comes back to Sarah, saying 'And then . . .' In this way Sarah can be helped through this supportive intervention to follow up her initial reflections (Heron 1989).

Questioning

Questions are verbal communications that initiate particular responses and can be used in a variety of ways to open channels of communication. Turney *et al.* (1976) point out that questions are not always asked simply to elicit an answer: they are often used to convey an underlying need of which the patient may or may not be aware. Turney *et al.* (1976) group questions into three different categories: *questioner-centred, respondent-focused* and *group activity*. Questioner-centred questions are used mainly to meet the need of the questioner, and may be employed to obtain information, to focus attention, to arouse or spark off interest and curiosity and to initiate social interaction. Respondent-focused questions, which involve discovering facts about the respondent and taking an interest in them, may help to identify difficulties and problems, to ascertain the feelings, opinions and beliefs of the respondent and to assess the extent of the respondent's knowledge. Group activity questions are used to stimulate discussion and dialogue among a group of individuals, as in for example a teaching environment or in a self-help group. Nursing takes advantage of many differing forms of questions in the day to day management of practice, often with little conscious awareness.

Questions, when used with intention and deliberation, provide numerous opportunities to deepen and enhance the caring relationship, enabling the development of an empathic bond between nurse and patient. Since they prompt the patient to go further with their exploration, questions have a catalytic potential, helping to draw out the reluctant or reticent patient in a facilitative manner (Heron 1989). They can, however, be overused and used in an interrogative manner, having the effect of creating a barrier.

Open questions

Open questions do not suggest a predetermined response and as such allow the respondent the freedom to answer in a number of ways. They are particularly useful in the use of counselling skills for exploring personal information (respondent-focused). Open questions tend to begin with how, when, where, or what, and are generally formulated in broad terms so as to initiate a flow of information. Open questions can be advantageous in that very little prior knowledge is required to formulate the question and yet a great deal of unexpected information may be precipitated. Examples of open questions in the context of nursing can be seen on page 42.

Closed questions

Asking closed questions limits the type of response that can be made, usually eliciting a simple but less than informative 'yes' or 'no' answer. They are often used to ascertain factual information, with the content and the response being dictated by the questioner (questioner-centred). Further types of closed questions are the selective question, in which the answer to the question is restricted by providing the respondent with a few alternatives, and the factual question. Factual closed questions are used frequently in nursing, for example in eliciting a history from the patient: 'Who is your next of kin?' – to find out facts: 'Are you on any medication?' – or to suggest possibilities: 'Would you prefer to have a bath or a shower?' In helping people to explore more of what they feel, however, closed questions are far less useful.

Leading questions

Where leading questions are used the question itself usually points to the preferred answer. Hargie *et al.* (1986) identify four types of leading questions: *simple leads, conversational leads, implication leads* and *subtle leads*. Simple lead questions, for example, are often set around a statement of fact: 'You won't be wanting any visitors this evening, will you?', 'It's definitely looking better, isn't it?

Probing questions

This type of question encourages expansion on previously made points. Probing questions may help in clarifying a problem and in eliciting examples of specific issues: 'Can you give an example of what might trigger off the vomiting?'

Affective questions

Affective questions ask the respondent to relate their feelings, referring to the subjective emotional state of the individual as opposed to the objective interpretation of facts. The nurse may need to guide the patient/family carefully to acknowledge and articulate their feelings, which can at times be difficult to access (an example is given on page 42).

Rhetorical questions

Rhetorical questions are not asked with the intention of receiving an answer; indeed at times the questioner may go on to provide the answer themselves, or use the question as a summary, before moving the patient on by asking a further question (again, see example below).

A dialogue may therefore run in this way:

Nurse: Are you in pain? (*closed question*)
Patient: Yes.
Nurse: Where do you feel the pain? (*probing question*)
Patient: In the same place, my lower back.
Nurse: Would you like to take something for it? (*closed question*)
Patient: Yes please.
Nurse: OK, I'll be right back.

Nurse: Have you been in hospital before? (*closed question*)
Patient: Yes.
Nurse: What was that like? (*open question*)
Patient: It was years ago, I don't remember much about it and I wasn't having surgery . . .

Nurse: Tell me about your eating habits? (*open question*)
Patient: I just seem to eat for the sake of it, almost always without thinking about it, especially when I am on my own. It has become a real problem now that I am pregnant. I know it's not good for the baby for me to be so overweight, but I can't seem to stop myself. It's like I don't have any control over it.
Nurse: So you haven't been successful in losing weight before (*rhetorical question*), and now you are concerned for your and your baby's health? (*closed question*)

Nurse: How do you feel about your wife having a mastectomy? (*affective question*)
Patient: I think she will manage, she's got a lot of fight in her.
Nurse: She's certainly a determined lady. How about you, how are you feeling about it all? (*affective question*)

Nurse: It is usual for a mother of your age to have this test. Are you happy to go ahead or is there anything else you would like to know about it? (*open question*)

Patient: I am a bit concerned, I don't want the baby to come to any harm.

Nurse: What is it in particular that concerns you? (*probing question*)

Patient: Someone told me that inserting the needle can lead to an abortion or cause some damage to the baby's brain. Is this true?

Nurse: You wouldn't want your mother to be present at the birth though, would you? (*leading question*)

Patient: Well . . . actually . . . she is my next of kin, and I would like her to be there . . . but if that would be a problem . . .

Nurse: Oh no, no, not at all.

Nurses use questioning skills constantly in their everyday practice, most notably in admitting the patient to a clinical area, or taking a history in primary care settings. Using questions in conjunction with some of the other listening skills already outlined can facilitate the development of a therapeutic relationship which goes some way to creating the conditions for healing to take place (Freshwater 2002). Once questions have been asked it is important that the nurse allows time for the patient to collect their thoughts and formulate their answer. This involves the nurse listening and paying attention. Sometimes it will be necessary to check that the question has been understood and the question may need to be rephrased. As previously mentioned, selective echoing of the patient's words may also be used as a form of question, as can skills such as paraphrasing and summarizing, in which the nurse can assess the degree of understanding that is being communicated.

Paraphrasing

Paraphrasing involves putting the patient's statements, thoughts and feelings into one's own words. By crystallizing the ideas and feelings of the patient the practitioner may not only demonstrate a degree of understanding of what has been said, but also act as a mirror to the patient's comments, allowing the patient to experience the impact of their words in the other person. When paraphrasing the nurse may either condense or expand what the patient has said, either way trying to capture the main meaning or feeling expressed by the patient's communication.

In the following example the nurse is responding to a patient who is having dialysis and waiting for a kidney transplant.

Patient: You would think I'd be used to this by now. Every time I come here I think it's going to get easier, but it never does. I still hate all the smells and sounds. I never have been very good in hospitals. At least I know a few faces here, but you know, it makes it harder that some people don't come back. I never know if the operations have been a success or not. It makes me wonder about mine.

Nurse: Even though you are a regular visitor here, it still feels hard being here. (*Here the nurse paraphrases the patient's words to encapsulate the feeling behind them.*)

Patient: Yes, in some ways I don't want to get used to it. I don't want to get used to the people either. It's too hard to cope with . . . when . . .

Nurse: When?

Patient: When everything is so uncertain for all of us . . .

Summarizing

Summarizing can prove to be a useful way of helping patients when they feel confused or stuck. It is also helpful for a nurse or health visitor when they feel they have gathered a lot of information and want to make sure they have understood the complexity of the patient's situation. The nurse can summarize at various points in the session, gathering the concerns that have been expressed and reflecting them back to the patient in a short summary. Picking out the main points from a fairly large amount of dialogue and condensing them into a short phrase can also help the patient focus on their main concerns, assessing the relative importance of each issue. This enables the patient to choose the direction in which they would like to go.

In this example the nurse is in conversation with a young girl who has just had a colostomy formed.

Patient: I don't think I will ever get used to it. It doesn't hurt anymore – if anything I am starting to feel better for the first time in ages. It just smells. That's the bit I hate: it smells all the time. I can tell that other people don't like it too. Even the nurses pull faces when they have to change it. No bloke is going to come within a mile of me.

Nurse: Sounds like you are really concerned about the effect this has on other people?

Patient: Well yes . . . what am I supposed to do? Of course my friends aren't going to say anything to my face; they are all really nice to me. But nobody likes the idea of having a bag on their stomach, let alone one what stinks and makes noises . . .

Nurse: Makes noises?

Patient: Yes, it does. Depending upon what I've been eating, it can be really bad. I mean I am still getting wind. Really sociable habit isn't it, emptying your bag and stinking the place out, or having really bad wind coming from your stomach. This is really going to go down well in a pub. My social life is really going to suffer.

Nurse: You are really worried about how you are going to carry on a normal social life, now that you have the colostomy; and you're anxious about managing the smells and the sounds in public places.

This example is perhaps a good place to begin to point out some of the distractions within a nursing context to using basic counselling skills effectively. Staying alongside the patient may not always be easy, with both nurse and patient encountering regular and varied distractions. One such distraction is that of the patient's medication. Certain medications may interfere with the ability of the patient to hear and understand what is being said to them. A patient who has been sedated pre- or post-operatively is not likely to be able to engage in a therapeutic encounter or remember it lucidly. Of course specific medical conditions (physical and psychological) also impair the patient's ability to remain focused on their concerns. Patients who are experiencing a lot of pain, or are confused or depressed, may find it hard to give the attention to themselves that a counselling type of situation demands. In the case of the patient with the new colostomy (above), anxiety levels might interfere with their ability to hear any assurances made by the nurse, as could smells and sounds. Nurses themselves may also struggle to hear what the patient is saying, distracted by their own inner thoughts and feelings.

An important consideration is when to use counselling skills. They are not necessarily appropriate, or indeed welcome when they are unsolicited. Patients seek help from nursing staff for all kinds of reasons, such as information, reassurance, advice, or just to have a conversation. Many practitioners would probably say there is no time at all for counselling and it is still not uncommon to hear practitioners justifying themselves when they are 'just talking' to their patients, as if it is not seen as a legitimate nursing activity. Occasionally, however, patients may ask a disguised question or indicate that they are distressed via other means.

Achieving basic empathy

What this chapter has described are the skills of accurate listening and responding. These skills are used with accurate listening skills to achieve an empathic rapport, and to develop an awareness of the uniqueness of each patient. If the nurse can step into the patient's world, albeit briefly, then empathy has been achieved, although the nature and degree of empathy experienced by the patient will be very much dependent on the relationship and the level of interaction attained.

Basic empathy is also associated with trust, power and control. I have referred already to issues of power that exist as much within the nurse–patient relationship as they do in other helping relationships. Active involvement of the user in their own healthcare is something that is receiving much publicity of late, with specific agendas being driven by user groups and the consumer voice. Counselling skills have the potential to move this agenda beyond the potential for tokenism to one in which the patient can experience an active alliance. Nurses using counselling skills are essentially involved in a cooperative partnership, rather than a competitive one. Nursing, like other professions, has traditionally been based on a unilateral model of caring. The move towards a joint activity such as is typical of most forms of counselling is not necessarily an easy one to make.

Empathy, personal and professional self

Basic empathy enables the nurse to relate to the patient more completely, viewing the person as a whole, rather than as an object. This more complete way of relating to the patient can be referred to as the I–Thou position (Buber 1958). The incomplete experience of the self and other is known as the I–It attitude. As Briant and Freshwater comment: 'The I–It attitude is one which the other person is never viewed as a whole being. It can never be the basis for a holistic relationship' (1998: 208). The I–It position is one that has been found to exist widely within nursing. Menzies-Lyth (1970), in her research into social systems, found that nurses view patients as objects as a way of coping with the intense anxiety that such intimate relationships cause. Nurses often manage high levels of distress and anxiety by relating both to themselves and to their patients as objects. The I–Thou approach to a relationship is based in equality, with one individual in her/his totality relating to the other in her/his totality. As I have already suggested this may be difficult to achieve within nursing due to the fiduciary nature of the relationship.

Summary

Nursing, like counselling itself, involves the formation of a meaningful relationship through the development of an effective interpersonal process. Efficacy is achieved through listening, the most human of all actions, which is an active process that involves all the senses, not just the ears. It is easy to take listening for granted and, through our own preconceptions, to fail to really listen. Gordon argues that, 'Listening is not a "technique" that can be taught'. It is, he says, 'an art or craft which can be developed only by practice. So listening is a stance, a position, an attitude that we can choose to take – or not'. He concludes that in order to listen 'we must really want to do it' (1999: 73). We listen not just to what is being said, nor simply to the content of the dialogue, but also to how something is being said. In addition the other person is not the only thing to which we listen, we listen too to the inner voice. Nurses will be able to respond in an appropriate manner if they have a sound grasp of the skills involved in accurate listening and are willing to use their own self-awareness to better understand the patient and themselves. Chapter 4 focuses on achieving a deeper under-standing of the nurse–patient interaction through the skills of advanced empathy.

Chapter 4

Sustaining the relationship

The skills of listening, exploring and clarifying described in Chapter 3 help create a climate in which the patient feels heard and respected and both the patient and practitioner experience a degree of trust. Through this interaction a number of concerns relevant to the patient's situation may have been raised. At this point the nurse might hope to enable the patient to achieve a greater understanding of some of the thoughts, feelings and issues that they have explored together. This requires that the relationship is simultaneously maintained and developed. The skills used in sustaining a therapeutic relationship while helping the patient to add depth to their concerns involve identifying links in what has been said, and at times encouraging the patient to take a broader view of their concerns.

These skills are used in addition to the skills of accurate listening. Indeed they rather depend on basic empathy as a foundation for moving the patient forward. As the patient expands in self-knowledge, depth and detail may precipitate hidden feelings and thoughts that can be experienced as threatening, or even overwhelming. It is at this point that the patient may also encounter some emotional tension and/or cognitive dissonance (Festinger 1957). When this happens patients are likely to protect themselves, using established patterns of defending themselves to resist challenges to their already formulated self-concept.

This chapter then concentrates on helping the nurse to acquire the skills necessary to help the patient piece together broad themes and patterns and where appropriate to develop new perspectives on their situation and on themselves. The counselling skills used in maintaining and deepening the therapeutic relationship are more psychologically intimate, and according to French 'represent a more intense, thorough and pointed look at the patient's concerns' than those of the exploration phase. He adds that in this phase of the work 'the counsellor becomes more of a verbal participant' and the relationship moves up a gear in intensity (1983: 183). Skills such as self-disclosure, challenging, immediacy and pattern identification are therefore discussed in this chapter and linked to the notion of advanced empathy. Exploration of the concepts of resistance and defences is undertaken in order to illustrate some of the dynamics that the practitioner may encounter as the therapeutic alliance deepens.

Advanced empathy

Described most simply, advanced empathy is the sharing of hunches with patients in a way that helps them to see their concerns more clearly. Hence advanced empathy is experienced when certain meaning is heard and implied but not yet openly expressed. In this sense advanced empathy confronts the patient, asking them to make the implicit explicit. The patient may not be wholly aware of the meaning implied within their interaction and as such might find advanced empathy somewhat unsettling. A further challenge presented by the move to advanced empathy is the subsequent deepening of the relationship.

Advanced empathy is often expressed through tentative interpretations and hunches that help the patient to see the bigger picture. Such interpretations open up areas that the patient is only vaguely aware of, or hinting at, and as yet unable to fully accept as part of their experience. Because such interpretations are (when accurate) based in the patient's experience, however, they resonate because the patient recognizes himself or herself in what is said.

Thus in the second phase of the therapeutic alliance the boundaries of the patient's self-awareness are stretched. French outlines ways in which the nurse may achieve advanced empathy, some of which are summarized below:

- identifying themes by tentatively suggesting trains of thought or trends, which run, like continuous threads through the dialogue. For example: 'You have mentioned your fear a number of times: is this something you would like to explore a bit more?'
- assisting the patient to the ultimate conclusions of what they have said. This may include future-oriented questions such as 'What do you imagine would be the worst thing that could happen if you don't continue with your medication?'
- pointing to potential links or bridges between apparently un-related thoughts, feelings and facts. For example: 'Do you see any way in which your fear of loneliness is related to your husband's illness?'
- restating words that the patient has said in vague, disjointed or confused terms, in a clear manner.

(adapted from French 1983)

The skills of advanced empathy include:

- challenging;
- immediacy;
- self-disclosure;
- dealing with resistance;
- offering alternative frames of reference;
- identification of themes and patterns (making links).

I briefly examine the counselling skills that can help to deepen an existing nurse–patient relationship.

Challenging

Challenging in counselling has several purposes. Among other things it aims to provide an accurate picture of the patient and their situation; to point out unacknowledged strengths and difficulties, and to encourage action or change. Burnard (1990)

drawing on the work of Heron (1989) and his six-category intervention analysis provides examples of issues on which the
patient might be confronted:

- direct feedback on behaviour, use of language, attitudes etc.;
- direct feedback on the effects of the other person's behaviour
  on self and others;
- challenging illogicalities and inconsistencies;
- challenging incongruities between what is said and the body
  language that accompanies it;
- challenging unaware, unconscious behaviour;
- drawing attention to contractual issues;
- drawing attention to rules or codes of contact.

(adapted from Burnard 1990: 129)

It should be noted that the aim of challenging is not accu-
satory, nor is it to make the patient feel small or told-off. A
challenge delivered by a caring person, and combined with the
core conditions of respect, congruence and genuineness (see
Chapter 1), will usually be well received, even if it is sometimes
painful.

Essentially, anything that invites individuals to examine
their behaviour, attitudes or beliefs in detail can be seen as challenging. This includes challenging strengths and successes that
the patient might let slip by or undermine; examining discrep-
ancies between the way patients view themselves and the way
they are viewed by the practitioner; challenging distortions and
projections; and challenging self-defeating behaviours. Egan
(1994) describes challenging as probably the most powerful and
most dangerous counselling skill. He suggests that a challenge
should be enough to evoke action in the patient without causing
them to feel cornered or trapped. In order to avoid phrases that
could lead to the patient feeling blamed or caught out, it is
advisable to frame observations in the form of open questions
that allow the patient a variety of response options. It is possible
that a patient may not immediately accept challenge but may
come back to it having given it some thought.

The following example illustrates how challenging unreal-
istic expectations or inaccurate self-belief needs to be done with
both sensitivity and positive regard:

Patient: What's the point anyway? I am sick of pretending that I will ever get out of this wheelchair. I'm a cripple and that's the end of it. I can't walk and I will never be able to again. I am not coming back to this clinic either.

Nurse: It sounds as if you are really fed up with putting in so much effort and seeing such little progress. I wonder if you expected more of yourself than is realistic?

[Alternative responses include: 'You've used the phrase "I can't" several times now. Can you help me to understand what you mean by this?' and 'Can I check something with you, are you saying that you can't walk or that you won't walk?']

In the following example Mark is reluctant to see that his intermittent drug taking is addictive or threatening in any way, but is constantly rationalizing his use.

Nurse: Mark, am I correct in thinking that you take ecstasy and speed every weekend?

Mark: Yeah, but I only take it at the weekend, never in the week, unless it's outside term time. I am not addicted, see; I don't use drugs in the week.

Nurse: When was the last time you were on a break from university and didn't take drugs?

Mark: Uhh . . . I don't take drugs all the time when I am off, mainly at the weekends . . . so it's hard to say . . . I only use soft drugs, the ones that aren't dangerous. I always get them from the same place . . .

Nurse: Mark, I notice that you are constantly justifying your use of drugs to yourself, almost as if you are trying to persuade yourself that you are not addicted and that it is a safe habit you have. I wonder . . . do you believe it yourself?

Offering alternative frames of reference

In Chapter 1 I outlined the person-centred approach to counselling, which clearly promotes a non-judgemental attitude towards the patient and their problems. When inviting the patient to view their problem and themselves differently the nurse verges on the edge of judgementality and as such is encouraged to consider carefully any alternative view proposed. In the nurse–patient relationship, just as in the counsellor–client relationship, the patient may feel unable to refute suggestions made by the nurse, viewing the nurse as the expert. In addition, the patient is to some extent dependent on the nurse for their care and may fear reprisals should they not agree with the practitioner's views. The skill in offering an alternative frame of reference lies in the nurse's intention, and in the phrasing of the suggestion, which always takes the form of an invitation to the patient. Examples of phraseology include: 'Is it possible that . . . ?' 'What is it like when I . . . ?'

Immediacy

Immediacy can be defined as the skill of discussing the relationship with the patient as it is in the moment. It is what Egan (1994) refers to as direct mutual talk. Thus it shifts the focus from the patient's problem to a better understanding of how both patient and nurse are behaving towards each other. Capturing the nuances of immediacy Egan (1994) denotes three slightly different layers to the skill, that of *general* relationship immediacy (how are *we* doing?), here and now immediacy (related to a *particular* event in the session) and self-involving statements (present tense personal responses to the patient).

Patients often present the very behaviour and feelings that they have difficulty with in the relationship with the practitioner. Thus the use of immediacy may point to the fact that a therapeutic alliance has or has not been created, that the rapport between the practitioner and patient is either very intimate or does not seem to be working. It may also highlight the existence of resistance and perhaps help to alleviate it. Immediacy is one way of working with patients who set up an interaction with the practitioner that is similar to the other relationships in their lives. This is where the psychodynamic concepts of transference and counter-transference help us to understand what may be going on.

Transference can be defined as the repetition by the patient of old child-like patterns of relating to significant people, such as parents, but now seen in relation to current significant figures, like a counsellor, nurse or doctor (Jacobs 1991). Counter-transference is defined as feelings that are evoked in the counsellor or practitioner by the patient (Jacobs 1991). Occasionally patients get stuck in the way they experience themselves and their lives, talking only about the past; use of immediacy and counter-transference feelings may help the patient to face how they feel just at that moment. There is of course the risk here that the practitioner's feelings get confused with the patient's, emphasizing the need for self-awareness and adequate support and supervision (see Chapter 6).

For example, the nurse who continually experiences strong emotions of anger and sadness when listening to this post-mastectomy patient might respond in the following way:

Patient: When I found out that my mammogram was dodgy I wasn't really concerned. I never really wanted to go for the mammogram anyway; it was my doctor that insisted I should have it done. I never have been one for checking up on myself. What will be, will be, I've always thought. I went more for my husband really.

Nurse: Listening to you, I find it difficult to know how you really feel right now.

Patient: Right now . . . well, I hadn't really thought about it . . .

[Note the patient responds to the feeling question from a cognitive stance.]

Immediacy can also be used to focus the direction of the relationship, paying particular attention to differences that might have a bearing on the work, such as cultural differences and gender-specific issues. Let us imagine that in the above scenario the nurse is male and is acutely aware at this point of conversation of his gender difference. Using immediacy the nurse may respond in any number of ways, one of which could focus on the 'here and now' encounter with the patient: I am wondering how it feels to be talking about this to me as a man right now?

Immediacy involves practitioners putting themselves on the line about their own feelings and what is going on; as such they are also confronting themselves. Thus immediacy is closely associated with self-disclosure.

Self-disclosure

Nurses disclose themselves to their patients indirectly each time they communicate with them, through movements, gestures, words or looks. Direct self-disclosure however is a skill that may be used by the practitioner intentionally and deliberately in the course of a therapeutic encounter. Self-disclosure is the art of sharing a personal experience with the patient, but with the aim of casting new light on the patient's situation and of creating a more trusting relationship. The latter is achieved as the practitioner demonstrates to the patient that they understand the patient's experience, and has perhaps been affected by similar events. Self-disclosure by the nurse not only demonstrates their willingness to trust the patient, but also begins to address the power imbalance that may be perceived in the one-sided sharing of private information.

Self-disclosure must however be used with discretion. Accurately and appropriately used it can be a positive and helpful way of bringing more of a human element to the nurse–patient association. One of the dangers of self-disclosure is that it takes the focus of concern away from the patient, and may even place the burden of the practitioner's problems on the patient. Hence while this phase of the relationship demands greater involvement from both parties, it is also important that the nurse does not invade or control the patient's space. 'Being over concerned with oneself is a natural human predisposition, but in order to be empathic it is necessary to suspend this persistent self-concern which has become a habit for most of us' (French 1983: 187).

The phenomenon of 'not realising how we affect others is also a common trait' (French 1983: 189), and is just as true of the nurse as it is of the patient. For example, Sarah is a 38-year-old single professional woman who is struggling to make connections with people following the death of her father four months ago. A health visitor who was recently bereaved might respond to Sarah saying, 'When my father died I found it really difficult to concentrate on other relationships for some time. I needed the space to grieve'. It is likely that this disclosure might open up the interaction with Sarah. However if the health visitor continues, 'My husband found it really difficult to understand what was going on for me, in fact I became really worried about our relationship . . .', then Sarah is more likely to feel brushed aside.

For Ted, a 50-year-old smoker who has been given an ultimatum – 'stop smoking or risk another heart attack' – the nurse might respond to his despair at his failed attempts by saying, 'I found that I stopped and started again a few times before I was really able to give up'. This response may on the one hand assist Ted in realizing that he has not failed, and that he, like other people in his situation (including health professionals), is struggling to control his craving. On the other hand, Ted might hear this response as a statement of the nurse's success, a sort of 'I have been able to manage this . . . you should be able to do the same', thus alienating him. Self-disclosure has to be done thoughtfully.

Egan (1994) cautions us to remain flexible in the application of self-disclosure, arguing that each patient is unique and as such demands a re-evaluation of the appropriateness of helper self-revelation. A useful question to ask of oneself when contemplating disclosure is 'Whose benefit is this for? Mine or the patient's?'

In Chapter 1 I began to outline some of the concepts originating in psychodynamic theories of the self. Of particular relevance to this phase of counselling are defence mechanisms, resistance, and, as already mentioned, transference and counter-transference.

Dealing with resistance

Resistance occurs when the patient mobilizes their resources against the nurse in order to thwart aspects of the helping relationship. Signs of resistance in the patient may include irrelevant comments or remarks, silence, or ignoring the practitioner's interventions. Resistance does not necessarily signal a negative relationship, and indeed early recognition and signalling to the patient may help relieve its negative effects. Freud (1915) believed that resistance was something to be worked through and overcome; this can often be accomplished by focusing on the empathic nature of the relationship.

Defence mechanisms are a healthy part of everyday life, enabling the individual to function in society. As French (1983: 184) notes:

The function of a mental defence mechanism is to protect individuals from the emotional pain of accepting truths or facts about themselves which they find intolerable. Were it not for defence mechanisms, most individuals would suffer such anxiety from emotional conflict that they would find it difficult to live a satisfactory and productive life.

One very common defence mechanism is that of projection. This involves ascribing ideas, feelings, behaviours and thoughts to another person, while not being aware that they also describe oneself. For example a frail elderly patient who is frustrated with her lack of independence says to her carer: 'You're fed up with me. I'm just a burden getting in your way all the time. Why don't you do away with me?' This may be an indication of the patient's own experience of being 'fed up' of relying on her carer, and a reflection of her own thoughts of ending her life.

Other common defences that may be found in clinical nursing situations are denial, rationalization and repression. Denial is often to be found in situations where patients are not willing or are unable to face a distressing reality, such as the death of a loved one; the realization of a terminal illness or the acceptance of a disfigurement. A patient might be heard to say: 'It's not so bad being in a wheelchair, at least I get a good seat in the cinema; and I was never any good at football anyway'. This appears to indicate both denial and rationalization.

Rationalization is in this case employed as a defence in order to alleviate anxiety or disappointment. Another defence, repression, censors unconscious material which can then manifest itself in slips of the tongue, lapses of memory and in dreams. Hence patients may forget important information regarding their health and treatment options, despite being advised of the appropriate facts on several occasions.

Awareness of defence mechanisms may be helpful to the nurse in their understanding of the patient, but it is not always necessary or helpful to point out to the patient their use of them.

Nurses also use defences, of course, to protect themselves in distressing and anxiety-provoking situations. This will be addressed in more detail in Chapter 7 where I describe the definitive work of Isobel Menzies-Lyth (1970, 1988). Nevertheless it is worth pointing out that patients can relate to the practitioner in all manner of ways, sometimes rendering it difficult for the practitioner to remain congruent and genuine, and so provoking the use of defences in the practitioner as well. In a notable study entitled *The Unpopular Patient* Stockwell (1972) found some patients were highly unpopular due to their deviance from the prescribed 'sick role' (Parsons 1966). The sick role demands that the patient adopts a dependent stance, accepts treatment unquestioningly and follows instructions. As Kirby and Slevin observe, however, patients who deviate from this expected role refuse 'to subsume his or herself to the prescribed sick role' (1999: 68). They go on to comment that this is only a problem for nurses if they are themselves absorbed in a prescribed inauthentic role. Nurses obviously have to suppress all kinds of negative feelings, so we can imagine a situation where the defence works less well, so that a nurse who is tired of hearing a patient's constant complaint and irritated with the patient who is repeatedly incontinent accidentally says 'It's no pleasure' instead of saying to the patient 'It's no trouble'!

Identifying themes and patterns

Enabling patients to identify themes and patterns that emerge in their responses is a crucial aspect of counselling that also applies in using counselling skills in nursing. Egan (1994: 183) suggests that thematic material might

> refer to feelings (such as themes of hurt, of depression, of anxiety), to behaviour (such as themes of controlling others, of avoiding intimacy, of blaming others, of overwork), to experiences (such as themes of being a victim, of being seduced, of being punished, of failing) or some combination of these.

The following example illustrates this:

> Deirdre has been caring for her elderly mother at home for the past five years, since her mother suffered a disabling stroke. Her mother attends a day centre two days a week to

give Deirdre some respite and time to care for her own family. On these days Deirdre is a volunteer at the local junior school, helping children with special educational needs. She was a nurse until 12 years ago, when she gave up full time work to look after her new daughter. In talking to the health visitor she reveals how tired she is, speaking of her disappointment in the quality of time she is able to give to her daughter and husband. The health visitor, having known Deirdre for some time, responds by reflecting, 'Caring for others seems to be something of a pattern in your life: you came out of nursing to care for your daughter and now you are caring for your mother. In the time that is put aside for you each week you volunteer to help others; and now you are worried about the quality of the care you give. It is as if you feel that what you are giving is not good enough'.

In summarizing Deirdre's situation the health visitor carefully brings together the theme of 'caring for others' with the concept of 'not being good enough', which is a characteristic that Deirdre has been expressing only vaguely up to now, but that the health visitor has been aware of for some time.

Summary

The skills involved in advanced empathy facilitate the communication of an understanding of the patient by the practitioner, and goes beyond the obvious words to the latent meaning of what has been said. This deeper level of communication can be challenging and fulfilling for both parties, requiring a degree of sensitivity, respect and mutual regard. Skills used in the development of advanced empathy are aimed at helping the patient to achieve a more accurate and dynamic understanding of the self. To this end it is important that the practitioner also has an awareness of himself or herself and of how they relate to particular aspects of specific patients. Before moving on to the third phase of the counselling process, it is essential that the patient has an opportunity to understand and accept something of the way they react to themselves and others, as well as to begin to realize the personal resources they possess, both used and unused.

In the next chapter I outline skills that are aimed at facilitating action based on this new understanding. These skills include divergent thinking, decision-making processes, goal setting and evaluation skills. The chapter also explores the role of teaching, advising and information giving within the nurse–patient interaction, including ways in which the practitioner can assist the patient to seek further support, or to accept the possibility of inaction.

Chapter 5

Facilitating change

When patients experience themselves as free from the forces that have been restraining them, they are able to contemplate action. It is at this point that the practitioner, using counselling skills, may assist the patient to mobilize their resources (internal and external) and develop a plan of action. This action plan can be divided into two main stages, thinking about the change and carrying it through. Each stage consists of smaller manageable objectives and is subject to ongoing evaluation and readjustment as action is implemented.

Building on the existing therapeutic alliance and using the patient's new insights the practitioner uses counselling skills to facilitate action based on new understanding, including divergent thinking, decision-making processes and evaluation skills. This chapter explores these skills in more detail and identifies the role of teaching, advising and information-giving within the nurse–patient interaction, including ways in which the practitioner may assist the patient to seek further support through referral. The ending of the therapeutic relationship also requires specific skills, some of which are addressed in the latter part of this chapter.

The skills that have been discussed so far have been concerned with relationship-building and enhancing the emotional well-being of the individual, carefully avoiding telling the patient what to do. Action-oriented skills are more directive and aim to change behaviour. Thus while the practitioner provides support and direction for the patient, this is done within a climate of commitment from the individual. This is particularly the case in specialist fields such as health promotion counselling. The Health of the Nation targets set by the Department of Health in 1992 have meant that many nurses are engaged in roles that aim to get people to change unhealthy behaviours into healthy ones (Sidell 1997). An example of a model of behavioural change is that of Prochaska and DiClemente (1984). This model has been very influential in alcohol counselling, and has been adapted in nursing to a variety of other settings. Nursing theorists have also developed models of care, which emphasize the patient's own role in taking control over their health needs (Orem 1971, 1990). However such models present the process of managing change as rather less complicated than may be experienced in reality. Change is very often unpredictable, fraught with difficulty and with the possibility of relapse. As Sidell (1997: 149) notes

> Helping people to change their behaviour is not just a matter of adopting the right counselling technique and learning the specific skills. Behaviour is firmly rooted in the psychological make up and located in social and cultural environments.

Naidoo and Wills (1994) contend that where change has been successful it is as a result of certain minimum conditions. They conclude that change:

- must be self-initiated;
- is often precipitated by other life events and is therefore salient;
- must not relate to a behaviour that is a fundamental coping strategy, making it difficult to resist and change;
- should not occur during a problematic or uncertain time as it can limit the individual's ability to adapt and change;
- is more effective where social support is available.

The degree to which the nurse is directive in the application of action-oriented skills will, of course, be dependent upon the individual situation and tailored to meet the needs of the specific alliance. Many of the skills identified within this chapter can be structured within a person-centred modality, that is by encouraging the patient through empathic responses to mobilize their resources. Even at this stage it is preferable for the intended actions to be decided by the patient, not imposed by the nurse.

Not all patients will be able to identify a measurable behavioural goal in relation to their problem; rather the nature of the patient's situation will dictate the intended outcome. For example, a patient dying of cancer may wish to work towards an acceptance of their condition, while a drug addict in withdrawal might have specific goals related to their rehabilitation programme. In addition patients with severe mental illness or under the influence of some medications are unlikely to be able to take part in the process of goal setting. The same is true of patients whose thought processes have been impaired due to the nature of their disease, as in for example neurological disorders. Whatever the intended outcome of the counselling it is important that the patient and the practitioner understand the purpose of the process and are committed to that purpose. The purpose, usually identified in the initial stages of the counselling process but referred to throughout the course of the alliance, may be used at this stage to assist in the setting of goals, and formulating action plans.

Action-oriented skills

In the third phase of the counselling process the practitioner aims to help the patient to initiate action, based on new understandings of themselves and their situation. In addition to the skills identified in previous chapters the nurse needs to draw upon further skills and knowledge, including knowledge of how behaviour is changed and maintained, as well as how to facilitate teaching and learning and setting realistic goals. The nurse and the patient work together to decrease forces that hinder change through identifying strengths and potential barriers to action. In Egan's (1994) terms the nurse is helping the patient towards action, and the patient's goal is to decide what action to take, if any, to resolve their problem. This can be achieved through a number of subskills and activities, such as identifying goals and behavioural objectives, force field analyses and decision balance sheets.

While patients may be working towards much-wanted change, they may also experience a sense of sadness once a decision to act has been reached. These and other emotions that are evoked at the ending of what is often a meaningful and intimate relationship require sensitive empathic responses so as to facilitate appropriate closure of the alliance. Both the practitioner and the patient need the opportunity to evaluate the process, the relationship and the outcomes.

A more detailed mapping of the skills is required to show how the process of change can be enabled, namely:

- divergent thinking;
- goal setting;
- problem solving;
- teaching/information giving;
- evaluation skills.

Divergent thinking

Divergent thinking can be described as thinking outside the rigid boxes into which we often place our thoughts. In contrast to convergent thinking, which generally assumes that there is one right answer, divergent thinking assumes that there is more than one way to manage a problem. This differs from the skills of phase two, in that while it is also concerned with offering alternative perspectives, the focus of the skill of divergent thinking is action.

Goal setting

While identifying long- and short-term goals can happen even before seeing how the problem can be tackled, it is often easier once the patient has a fuller understanding of themselves and their situation. It is worth spending time with a patient assisting them to make a list of their goals, helping them to break them down into shorter- and longer-term components. Components of goal setting include an indication of intention from the patient, that is how they want to act; working towards a general statement of what the patient wants to do; defining and refining the goal into a realistic and accomplishable aim. One way of doing this is to encourage the patient to brainstorm things which they think would help them move forward. The nurse can use this opportunity to ask clarifying questions to assist in the goal-setting process. Sometimes short-term goals can only be outlined once long-term ones have been made more explicit.

Once such a list of goals has been established the patient can be asked to arrange the identified actions in order of priority; in this way a hierarchy of needs can be outlined. The nurse plays an important role in ensuring that the patient identifies goals that are not only achievable, but can be achieved sooner rather than later. These short-term enabling goals provide positive feedback to the patient, acting as 'positive reinforcers' and encouraging the patient to continue with their progress.

Positive reinforcement is based on Skinner's operant conditioning theory (1953). It is achieved through systematic reinforcement of healthy desired behaviours, strengthening adaptive behaviours, and ignoring unhealthy behaviours until they eventually become extinct. Positive reinforcement is used in everyday relationships, and is an inherent part of both nursing and of the counselling process; as Hough points out 'empathy, warmth, genuineness, praise, attention and listening, can be viewed as methods of reinforcement for clients' (1994: 137). However, in action-oriented approaches to counselling, the practitioner may use positive reinforcers more explicitly. Indeed in some clinical nursing situations desired behaviours are rewarded with privileges and gifts. Examples of this can be seen in psychiatric nursing where patients with anorexia nervosa are rewarded with privileges for maintaining or increasing their weight (see Skinner 1953; Richards and McDonald 1990; and Trower *et al.* 1990 for a more detailed exploration of positive reinforcement and how it links to token economy systems).

Goal setting is not an easy task, since very often patients set proposals for action in vague or woolly terms rather than in precise objective terms. French, drawing on the work of Mager

(1962), notes that 'behavioural objectives should state the goal in terms of what the client will be able to do to indicate that his goals have been achieved' (1983:192). Mager (1962) clarifies three components of good behavioural objectives, stating that they should: identify and name the overall behavioural act; define the conditions under which the behaviour is to occur; and decide how to measure minimal acceptable performance. Thus goals need to be:

S specific;
M measurable and variable;
A appropriate;
R realistic;
T time oriented.

For example Margaret, a 43-year-old single professional woman, has recently had a mastectomy. She was a keen athlete and swimmer prior to her surgery and was totally devastated when she discovered that the lump in her breast was malignant. In the period following her recovery she was able to talk about her future with the specialist breast care nurse. Throughout the relationship Margaret had been particularly concerned about her ability to swim again. This was her main social network and she belonged to a swimming club where she had many friends. She identified the two main issues as linked to pain and discomfort and, more importantly, to body image. As Margaret and the practitioner were working towards devising an action strategy, the nurse helped Margaret clarify her goals.

Margaret's main goal was to be able to swim comfortably again without feeling too self-conscious and without avoiding people. The nurse encouraged Margaret to break this goal down into a number of intermediate objectives, which included finding a suitable swimming costume with a breast prosthesis in which Margaret could feel safe to move freely, wearing the swimming costume in the house to get used to the range of movement permitted, and attending a swimming club social event in the evening without swimming. However, it was also important that the objectives attended to the emotions associated with the intended actions. Margaret was very unsure of how she would feel about exposing her body in a public place and felt fearful of how other people might see her. She was describing her own distaste at seeing her chest wall as well as experiencing a sense of shame and embarrassment. Thus action goals need to be feeling-oriented as well as thinking and behaviour-oriented. For example Margaret might aim to feel confidence in her body, as opposed to feeling ashamed and embarrassed.

This step by step approach, similar to the process of desensitization, can act as a framework for the patient to try out old skills within a new context. Desensitization, rather like positive reinforcement, is also based on classical conditioning techniques. It is often used to enable patients to deal with irrational fears and phobias and crippling anxiety. This was the case with Jenny, who had recently been diagnosed with diabetes mellitus. Jenny had been prescribed insulin to stabilize her blood sugar. However she had a needle phobia and was in a complete panic every time her insulin was due. During her time in hospital she had hidden in the lavatory and refused to come out, sobbing that she couldn't bear injections. Hence Jenny's diagnosis of being an insulin-dependent diabetic was particularly painful. The practice nurse within Jenny's GP surgery worked with Jenny on a desensitization hierarchy that listed several small objectives, and an overall goal of Jenny being able to inject herself with insulin. Progressive relaxation techniques were used as an integral part of the process, so that Jenny learned a skill that helped to master anxiety.

Obviously, as in Margaret's case (in which her fear of being exposed in public was perfectly rational) Jenny's fear of injections could be understood, but there are instances when a patient's fear and anxiety appears to be irrational. One such instance is Peter, who despite many diagnostic tests and procedures was convinced that he had a brain tumour. He had an absolute fear of the disease and refused to believe that his test results were within normal ranges. The resultant anxiety meant that Peter was unable to concentrate on his work, was not sleeping well and had no appetite, all of which of course contributed to him feeling unwell, thereby perpetuating his anxiety. The community psychiatric nurse working with Peter to help him with his anxiety and fears enabled Peter to identify that he was most anxious when he was on his own, and particularly in bed at night. In this case the work focused on getting Peter's anxiety to a manageable state so that he might be able to explore any underlying issues related to his fear. In this way goals are constantly revisited and amended in light of the patient's current needs.

Problem solving

It could be argued that counselling is a process that aims to help the client make decisions for themselves. According to French (1983) one way of interrupting the decision-making process is to be too directive as a counsellor and nurse. He argues that 'if one makes decisions for the client or presents ready-made solutions to problems, not only does this take away the impetus of decision making by the client, but it is also unlikely to suit them as an individual' (1983: 196). Thus the nurse needs to find alternative ways of encouraging the patient to come to their own decisions, while simultaneously offering support and guidance in line with their specialist knowledge and expertise.

Force-field analysis is a technique designed to enable an individual to understand the internal and external forces that influence the decision-making process. Having identified goals the patient can be encouraged to name the forces that will facilitate them and those that will restrain them. The aim is to work on decreasing the effect of the restraining forces and increasing the effect of the facilitating factors. Thus force-field analysis is linked to problem-solving with 'facilitating forces overcoming restraining forces in pursuit of success' (French 1983: 194).

An example of a force-field analysis is one that was completed by a patient awaiting a knee replacement, who had chronic chest infections and serious breathing difficulties due to prolonged and excessive smoking. The surgeon agreed to perform the surgery as soon as the patient was well enough both to endure the procedure and to give herself the best chance of a speedy recovery. She worked with the health promotion nurse to stop smoking and began to identify some of the restraining and facilitating forces. As the patient started to formulate her force-field analysis the nurse was able to reassess the patient's motivation for change, both intrinsic and extrinsic, getting a sense of where the main force of the change lies (see Figure 5.1).

Internal World	Internal World
Hinders	Helps
1 It's my treat, I enjoy it. 2 It's time to myself after the children have gone to bed. 3 I have tried to give up before and not succeeded.	1 My health is suffering, I have had two chest infections and I need the surgery on my knee. 2 I want to be able to walk better. 3 I owe it to myself; I don't feel good about myself at the moment.
External World	External World
Hinders	Helps
1 I go outside with others to smoke at work various points in the day. 2 I enjoy smoking when I go out for a drink. 3 My husband smokes.	1 Judith has just given up and is trying to encourage me. 2 Cigarettes are so expensive I would be much better off. 3 I will be able to have my surgery knowing that I have done my best to speed up my recovery.

Figure 5.1   Force-field analysis

Teaching and learning

As previously mentioned, the process of change may involve the patient learning different ways of responding or behaving. As such it is often the case that patients can learn new skills while engaged in the counselling process. Teaching is a part of every-day role for many nurses, whether this is through helping patients to understand the nature of their illness, teaching social skills, training in coping after discharge, demonstrating self-care, recommending activities in daily living, or teaching students new skills and concepts. When using teaching skills within the context of a counselling relationship it is important for the nurse to remind himself or herself of the nature of the nurse–patient dyad. The dependent nature of the relationship means that teaching can be a potential source of control and power, with the patient taking information from the nurse uncritically and without question. Where the nurse is teaching practical skills as part of the therapeutic process, for example in teaching a young first-time mother how to bathe her baby, care should be taken to engender confidence, independence and esteem within the patient. In the teaching of life skills it is preferable for the nurse to *show* rather than to *tell* the patient how to change. Role modelling provides one such framework for teaching both practical and psychosocial life skills.

Life skills are self-help skills which enable individuals to help themselves. They are aimed at empowering rather than weakening or undermining the patient, and can be focused on feelings and thoughts and/or on observable actions. One example of life skills is assertiveness training. This teaches patients to interact more effectively and comfortably with others, and can be taught on an individual or group basis. Patients who lack confidence in certain social situations can be taught to acquire the necessary skills to cope with life's challenges and difficult situations.

Information giving

Patients are sometimes unable to proceed to action because they lack the information necessary to move forward. Giving information and dispelling misinformation is a way of helping the patient to make well thought-through decisions. Providing the patient with specialist knowledge or assisting them in knowing where to find it may help the patient to see their situation in a different light and thus provide a basis for action (Egan 1994). Egan argues that information-sharing skills are challenging as they can compel the patient to see themselves and their situation quite differently. For this reason he urges a sense of caution and tact when using information-sharing skills. Information provided should be clear, relevant and without preconceived judgement. For example when helping Anne, a 49-year-old mother of two, to make a decision about her recently confirmed pregnancy, it was important that the midwife working with Anne provided her with unbiased facts and evidence concerning the potential risks associated with late pregnancies. This information would ultimately affect Anne's decision and how she lived with the consequences of that decision. Information-giving differs from offering advice and should not be confused with the latter, especially since telling the patient what you would do in a specific situation is seldom well received.

Evaluation

Nursing practice is based on a cyclical process that should be informed by constant evaluation. In counselling too evaluation brings about a reappraisal of the initial problem and of further areas for exploration. Ongoing evaluation provides an opportunity for the practitioner and the patient to explore what is happening and to appraise what has been achieved, and what therefore might be done next. A final evaluation provides a sense of completeness and is a point at which both nurse and patient can learn from each other. When the nurse and patient have been working together for some time it is possible that the original reason for engaging in the process has faded into the background as other more significant themes begin to emerge, so it is useful in a final evaluation to review the journey that has been taken. This is most often done through a review of the initial contract (contracting is addressed in more detail in Chapter 6).

Measuring success is notoriously difficult in counselling, particularly when viewed from the positivist viewpoint of evidence-based practice. It may be relatively easy, for example, to see a difference when using counselling skills to help someone change a behaviour, such as stopping smoking. It is less easy to measure the benefit to someone of being allowed to talk through uncomfortable feelings and emotions related to their illness in a safe environment, although the difficulty evaluating this certainly does not mean that it is not to the patient's benefit.

Ending the relationship

The endings of relationships are important and can be surprisingly difficult to deal with, for both the practitioner and the patient. The process requires sensitivity and self-awareness on the part of the practitioner. Each patient has a different experience of the therapeutic relationship and this, together with past experience of loss, tends to affect the ability of the patient to engage with the ending. Some counselling work is time-limited and as such the ending is determined from the beginning. In other nursing situations the length of the therapeutic work is defined by how long the patient is in hospital, or is receiving treatment. Where possible the patient's readiness for ending is assessed and negotiated mutually, to enable learning achieved during the counselling to be consolidated, and feelings associated with the ending to be expressed.

Whatever the situation, it is important to prepare the patient for the ending of the relationship. This can be done by referring clearly to it and by referring to the other losses that are occurring as the patient changes (such as the loss of the old self) and the relationship closes (and the loss of a particular kind of relationship). The process of disengagement also involves planning the ending, since this allows time for any unfinished business to be addressed. The practitioner's ability to model healthy letting go, and to work with loss in a positive way, is crucial to the satisfactory closure of the relationship. This also demands a deep awareness of the practitioner's own experiences of loss and any difficulties there may be with letting go.

Referral

Recognizing one's limitations is an essential part of any professional practice; inability to do so (or refusal to do so) can prove harmful to the patient. An important part of using counselling skills is knowing when to refer a patient to another source in order that they may be helped further, beyond what the nurse practitioner can achieve. Nurses working in a variety of settings have contact with a number of multiprofessional agencies and are often well placed to direct the patient to appropriate resources. The nurse should not see referral as a failure, but as the best form of help that the nurse can offer at that time. There are many reasons why a nurse might refer a patient to another source, some of which include:

- the patient does not respond to the offers of help by the nurse;
- the nurse does not have the time and capacity to work with the patient;
- the patient needs specialist advice or treatment;
- the patient may be more effectively helped by another;
- the patient needs intensive psychotherapy;
- the patient dislikes the nurse/the nurse dislikes the patient.

The counselling skills identified in phases one and two of the process are useful in dealing with the issue of referral sensitively, tactfully and empathetically.

Summary

Many of the patients with whom nurses deal are not physically fit, may be confused and fatigued, and in situations of physical and psychological dependence. Some of them will view the counselling process itself as sufficient action, and indeed in many cases it is. The opportunity for the nurse to use the counselling skills that they possess does not necessarily mean 'doing' anything, but being available.

Furthermore Egan (1994) reminds us that some patients, despite doing well in analysing problems, and in identifying reasonable strategies, goals and action plans, choose not to change. His point is that it is the patient's choice, and it may be that a patient who chooses to remain the same, does so from a more informed position. For those who are committed to changing a behaviour or pattern, however, the skills in this phase of the counselling process provide a structure within which the practitioner and the patient may together plan and implement change. As in all aspects of counselling the practitioner is challenged to maintain an awareness of their own needs and concerns in order to best support the patient to make their own decisions.

This work brings its own rewards, as patients value the opportunity to speak about their deeper fears and feelings, and in some cases make decisions and take actions which enable them to take the next steps in their recovery or in their adjustment to their situation. Inevitably using counselling skills to work with people at greater depth, like nursing itself, is an arduous task however, and one which cannot be carried out without the support of others. A nurse should also be willing to seek help in order to realize their own limitations and to reflect upon their work and their relationships with different patients. Chapter 6 attends further to the issue of self-awareness, focusing on the professional and ethical concerns associated with using counselling skills; topics such as boundary concerns, ethical issues, confidentiality and record-keeping are discussed in the context of clinical supervision and reflective practice.

Chapter 6

Professional considerations

One of the main purposes of using counselling skills in nursing is to enable the patient to recognize and explore feelings, thoughts and behaviours in greater depth. This can only be achieved in an environment in which the patient feels safe enough to do so, one that is free from criticism and judgement and has clear physical, professional and personal boundaries.

Providing time and space for patients to understand and clarify their problems and make meaningful choices of their own is a complex process, whether this is listening to a patient's fears about waking up from an anaesthetic, taking their worries seriously, or facilitating access to appropriate information about natural childbirth therefore enabling informed decisions to be made. The skill of the helper is to create an environment that can facilitate this process. This chapter addresses some of the personal, physical and professional boundaries that need to be considered, so that an environment conducive to the application of counselling skills can be fostered.

The use of counselling skills within a work environment also has professional, ethical and personal implications. Clinical supervision has been promoted as a method of ensuring safe and accountable practice in nursing (UKCC 1996). While various attempts have been made to define and describe clinical supervision, with an emphasis on standards, quality of care, patient safety and staff support, to date its implementation has been patchy and inconsistent. This chapter attends to the practice of clinical supervision within a profession that draws heavily upon counselling skills, emphasizing the professional issues that merit consideration within this specialist context. Topics such as boundary issues, ethical concerns, confidentiality, record-keeping, and the impact of future developments in nursing are also discussed.

Ethical concerns

There is little doubt that both nursing and counselling are professional practices that rely heavily upon the integrity of the individual practitioner. The code of practice for nurses, midwives and health visitors (UKCC 1992) and the duty to care are based on the four prima facie principles of ethics that have been developed over time, and which, it is argued, cut across all ethical, moral and political perspectives (Beauchamp and Childress 1983). These are:

- the principle of autonomy;
- the principle of beneficence;
- the principle of non-maleficence;
- the principle of justice.

While these ethical principles act as 'ideals' for health professionals in the administration of their daily tasks, there are often conflicting values in the application of such principles to everyday nursing practice. The two central tenets in nursing are to do good (beneficence) and to avoid harm (non-maleficence). Taking the example of health promotion Jones and Cribb (1997) discuss how some practices that health professionals engage in, which aim to improve the health of the patient, may also do damage to some people. Examples include encouraging the uptake of immunizations that carry the risk (albeit small) of side effects.

The principle of autonomy relates to the rights of people to determine their own lives and to have freedom of choice. This principle raises serious concerns about the legitimate right of practitioners to intervene and persuade people to take a particular course of action. Here again respecting autonomy creates dilemmas for those involved in promoting health, namely all health professionals. As Jones and Cribb (1997: 95) comment

> If the client makes a choice that the professional considers is harmful, the health professional may be torn between respecting the client's autonomy and doing good and avoiding harm. The temptation may be to persuade the client to act differently but if a major principle is freedom of choice it must be questioned whether and when there is any legitimate right to intervene or persuade people to a particular course of action.

It follows then that nurses, midwives and health visitors may find themselves in difficult situations, such as having to support individuals to make decisions that might conflict with the principles that underpin the UKCC (1992) code of ethics and practice. When a patient, despite being given all available information, makes a choice to act in a manner that is potentially detrimental to their well-being, such as choosing not to have diagnostic tests, discharging themselves from hospital, continuing to drink alcohol against medical advice, or refusing treatment, the nurse has little choice but to respect the individual's autonomy – except, that is, where the patient is mentally ill and is deemed to be a risk to themselves or others. Where there is doubt about the individual's ability to manage for themselves the principles of beneficence and maleficence override the principle of autonomy.

Ewles and Simnett (1995) take this debate further, examining the clash between the health professional's values and the cultural values of the patient. Using the example of hypertension they note that while lowering a patient's blood pressure may be the most important thing to a doctor, drinking beer in the pub may be more important to the overweight unemployed patient. Who is to say which set of values is right? The principle of autonomy is also linked to the notion of confidentiality, and the question of how much to tell a patient, or how much of what a patient tells you can be disclosed. These and other issues may need to be talked about in the process of negotiating a contract with the patient.

When using counselling skills as a part of nursing practice practitioners may find themselves in situations where they experience not only conflicting values and beliefs, but also dissonance around ethical and moral practices within healthcare itself. While this is not the place to enter into a debate around such concerns as equity in provision of care (linked to the principle of justice), ethical principles lie at the heart of both counselling and nursing. As such practitioners are urged to come to understand their own decision-making processes. There are a number of models to assist nurses in their ethical decisions; Seedhouse (1988) for example developed an ethical grid to enable practitioners to reflect systematically on their caring practices. More recently Johns (1998) has formulated an ethical mapping grid to assist in the processes of reflective practice (this is outlined in more detail in Chapter 7). While the benefit of hindsight is valuable, reflective practice does not only occur after the event. Using foresight and experience the nurse can, for example, introduce the concept of boundaries and limits through the negotiation of a contract.

Negotiating a contract

Prior to starting a relationship that is based on the use of counselling skills it is important to discuss the aims, goals and expectations of both parties. Failure to do this can lead to dissatisfaction for both patient and practitioner. When things go wrong in counselling it is often due to the contract not being sufficiently clear. A contract can be divided into the following areas:

- boundaries and limits;
- accountability and responsibility;
- aims, goals and preferred process.

The boundary issues focus the attention of the practitioner and the patient on certain questions regarding both the practicalities of the counselling work itself, and the legal and ethical responsibilities involved in a therapeutic relationship, some of which include:

- where will the meetings take place;
- at what time;

- how frequently;
- how will the work be evaluated;
- how will confidentiality be maintained;
- what should be documented;
- what are the rights and responsibilities of all participants.

Professional boundaries

Boundaries and limits

The term boundary is commonly used in counselling, and is one of particular significance as it emphasizes the importance of setting limits. It refers to issues such as confidentiality, record-keeping and time management.

Confidentiality

Although confidentiality is basic to counselling one might question whether counselling can ever be guaranteed to be a totally confidential activity. Can it really be said that there are no circumstances when confidentiality should be overridden? Within nursing practice there are also issues of concern related to the assumptions that confidentiality is a clear-cut issue (Dilworth 2000). When working with a patient in a therapeutic manner it is not sufficient enough to tell him or her that what is discussed can be totally confidential. Rather like counsellors, who are bound by their own code of ethics for practice (BACP 1998), nurses are bound by the United Kingdom Central Council (UKCC 1992) code of conduct, which clearly outlines the limits to confidentiality. However, like all codes of practice, the UKCC discusses these issues in a very general manner, leaving room for individual interpretation and contextual application. It might be thought that if the nurse utilizing counselling skills adopts the code of ethics and practice for those using counselling skills in their work (BACP 1999) high standards of confidentiality must be expected, but these standards have to be contextualized within the practitioner's primary role, that of nurse, midwife or health visitor. It is not unusual in this situation for practitioners to experience role conflict, something that is discussed below.

Patients, including all patients undergoing treatment within a professional setting, should be made aware of the limits of confidentiality. For those patients who are working with the practitioner in a more structured counselling relationship the limits of confidentiality should be discussed during the first phase of the counselling process. It is not possible for the nurse to promise confidentiality in advance of a disclosure from a patient; it is therefore preferable to deal with such concerns early on. A patient may ask the nurse, 'Can I tell you something private without you telling my doctor? Promise not to say anything?' The nurse will need to think carefully before answering such a question. One possible response might be to say, 'I can't promise that I won't tell your doctor, but what I can promise is to speak with you first if I feel it is important to talk to anyone else'. The practitioner may also want to make the patient aware of the system of support that the practitioner has, the referral system, other agencies available to support the patient, and how information is recorded. Where a nurse is clear about the limits of the confidentiality he or she will feel more confident in the counselling role, and this in turn will impact the developing alliance.

Record-keeping

Keeping notes and records of patient care is central to the nursing process and needs to be taken into consideration when using counselling skills in a work context. Some patients may be sensitive about information that could go into records and may therefore influence future decisions about their treatment. Indeed many patients are still concerned about both the stigma attached to counselling and receiving support of a psychological nature, particularly where they are linked with referrals to a psychiatrist or other similar services. In relation to record-keeping the same legal principles apply as with any other record. The patient has the right to access any records that have their name on them (Bond and Holland 1998).

The question of if, what and where to record notes pertaining to counselling within nursing is one that still requires some development. The nurse may add to the existing patient care plan, but once again must be mindful of the concerns around confidentiality. For those patients who are hospitalized or living in residential homes, records are often kept near the patient's bed space, meaning that visitors, carers and other health workers can access them. This is also true for those patients who are being visited at home, who are usually the custodians of their own progress records. When considering what to write it is worth reflecting on the purpose of the records. Whose agenda are they serving? What they are for? Are they a working document or purely a legal obligation? Often a note of the date and time of the meeting, with a brief outline of the area discussed, will suffice.

There are times when the practitioner may feel a moral duty to pass certain information on. The main justification for a breach of confidence is where the life of the individual (or the life of another) is at risk. For example if the mother of a severely disabled child, whose quality of life is seriously being questioned, indicates her plans to help the child to die, the practitioner is under an obligation to discuss this information with others. However, where this is felt to be necessary, it should be done, if possible, in negotiation with the patient, who should be informed of the likely outcome of any information that is passed on. Thus prior to using counselling skills within their everyday practice, practitioners need to familiarize themselves not only with the relevant professional legal liabilities and responsibilities and local policies. They should also have access to information about local and national resources, referral systems and patients' rights. This is never more pertinent than in the current climate of user and carer involvement in health care (DoH 1998, 1999).

Physical boundaries

Settings, time and place

The setting in which counselling takes place is a fundamental consideration and requires considerable forethought, not least because many of the individuals with whom nurses, midwives and health visitors are in contact are not only in unfamiliar territory, but are often already located within alien and disorientating settings, with their daily routines disrupted. Some patients are of course visited in their own homes, but those patients classified as the 'worried well' do not always refer themselves to the GP surgery. More and more patients are seeking advice from health professionals via telephone helplines such as NHS Direct and walk-in centres. This particular development has implications for the boundaries and limits of counselling skills, not least the influence of the counselling setting on the therapeutic relationship.

The physical environment

The physical setting that I wish to outline, for the purposes of developing a safe and trusting environment, is the ideal, and perhaps also idealistic; in reality there are many constraints placed upon both the practitioner and the patient in finding both the time, space and place for meaningful conversations to take place. The patient's own physical well-being and health tends to dictate where and when counselling can take place. For example a patient who has recently undergone major surgery, and is sited in a hospital ward in a bay with three other people, may not wish to talk in any great depth about their fears and concerns. Neither do curtains afford the best protection and privacy for the individual. However, beds are often wheeled around the clinical areas for physical tests and treatments, and where possible this should also be considered if a distressed patient requires a more private environment in which to talk. This is of course difficult in a situation where space is at a premium, where even sick patients find themselves lying in corridors waiting for more receptive and appropriate surroundings.

Similarly, the individual's home is not necessarily conducive to clear and creative thinking or the expression of bottled up emotions. Children or partners may be present; the telephone, television and music can be distracting. Again, where possible the patient should be offered the chance to meet the practitioner in a private room, perhaps within the GP's surgery. Often patients are afforded privacy in the practitioner's own office or in a room set aside for teaching. The room need not be large or lavishly furnished, but it is crucial to minimize noise and other distractions, such as interruptions from colleagues and on call pagers.

The provision of a suitable environment conveys a message to the patient that they are valued and that what they have to say matters. It also reduces the levels of stress for the practitioner if they are able to work in reasonable surroundings and give themselves the best chance of being an effective counsellor. The setting aside of time specifically for the purpose of attending to a patient's needs is not easily managed within a busy work schedule, and it therefore requires forward planning. This not only enables the practitioner to manage their time better, but also provides the patient (and practitioner) with a sense of structure. Meetings may take place on a one-off basis or more frequently over a sustained period of time. Nurses visiting patients in their own homes can opt to meet with their patients once a week for up to one hour, but it is unlikely that the practitioner will be able to provide any longer than an hour in any one meeting. It is actually unusual in counselling situations to offer sessions over 50 minutes long. More importantly, the nature of the patient's illness will determine the individual's ability to concentrate and make effective use of the time available. Fifty minutes is a good period of time even for the most healthy of individuals to focus, and with weak, tired, or stressed patients a shorter time is probably preferable. What is helpful, however, is to give the patient an indication at the start of how long the practitioner can be there.

The duration of the counselling work is also very much dependent on the individual situation; both short-term and long-term counselling relationships may be formed given the variety of contexts within which practitioners work. A health promotion practitioner may work with a patient who is trying to manage a lifestyle change for four to six sessions, while a Macmillan nurse caring for a patient in their own home may continue to work with the individual and their family over a number of months.

Thus far I have referred to counselling interventions that are planned and arranged. The opportunity to support a patient using counselling skills frequently presents itself in all manner of unplanned and unpredictable clinical situations: for example, escorting a patient to another department, performing a dressing, or weighing a baby. Nurses are adept at thinking on their feet and responding rapidly to dynamic events. Therefore nurses are well placed to integrate their counselling skills with the skills they have gained and refined in the management of their daily practice. Nevertheless, consistency is central to the development of a safe and trusting therapeutic relationship.

Maintaining consistency and constancy, while important to the development of a trusting counselling relationship, is problematic within nursing contexts. One example of this is that many practitioners are working shift patterns, which in itself is a challenge, but it can also mean that the nurse is away from the clinical area for several days at a time. It is not just the practitioner's schedule that has to be taken into account, since when working with patients who are unwell, on medication and even dying, the nurse and patient need to determine the timing of meetings carefully. For example, if a patient undergoing radiotherapy experiences nausea and tiredness following their treatment, it is wise to time the meetings between treatments rather than directly afterwards or before them.

Telephone counselling

Given that telephone and Internet counselling is becoming more commonplace it needs to be mentioned, although more detailed information about this can be found in the Appendix at the back of this book. While telephone consultations afford the caller a degree of anonymity, safety and control, they can be more taxing for the practitioner who has to respond to the caller without the aid of any visual clues. As a result the practitioner risks making assumptions about the patient, not least in regard to age, race and physical condition. Telephone counselling can move very fast, partly because of the greater readiness to express negative feeling. The nurse receiving and managing telephone calls to helplines is challenged to monitor their own and the caller's use of tone, volume, vocabulary, pace and pitch so as to facilitate attunement and empathy. Hence the concept of accurate listening takes on a slightly different dimension. While many of the skills discussed in previous chapters can be adapted to telephone counselling, the use of silence is particularly difficult, sometimes propelling the practitioner into a flurry of interrogation. As the patient is unable to see the reaction they are evoking in the practitioner, the nurse may instead want to assure the patient that they are still listening, perhaps by saying, 'I am here if you want to say anymore'.

Personal boundaries

Role conflict

Health care professionals have several roles, including teacher, carer, manager, supervisor, mentor, administrator and researcher. Successfully combining all these roles alongside that of counselling is both complicated and simple – simple, in that counselling skills can be used in many everyday situations, from managing a colleague's yearly appraisal to supporting a student through a practical assessment. However, the practitioner's ability to combine the different and occasionally conflicting roles of nurse and counsellor can lead to role confusion. Where a nurse may take it for granted that it is acceptable for them to make physical contact with a patient whom they have only recently met, a counsellor will generally experience much more caution around the question of touch. A nurse using counselling skills, having undertaken some training in counselling, is likely to find themselves more conscious of their body language and the way in which they use their physicality with their patients. This is not necessarily a difficulty, but it can nevertheless cause some cognitive dissonance.

Self-awareness

Development of self-awareness is a vital part of any counselling practice or training. Self-awareness can be achieved through a variety of ways, including basic counselling training, personal counselling, bibliotherapy, reflective practice and clinical supervision. The practitioner is expected to recognize their own personal values, beliefs and prejudices as well as their own emotional and physical needs. As indicated earlier distractions to being fully present with the patient can come from inside the practitioner as well as from external sources. They may appear in the form of prejudice, passing judgement, clashes of values or the nurse's own emotional needs. Self-awareness involves exploration of one's own personal motivations, including the motivation for caring and counselling. It is also closely linked to the skill of self-disclosure (see Chapter 3), which should be in the interests of helping the patient to achieve deeper self-understanding or to assist in self-exploration. Self-awareness enables the nurse to be selective and appropriate in the use of self-disclosure.

A further aspect of self-awareness is the role it plays in helping practitioners to monitor their levels of stress and coping, recognizing when they are reaching their limits and when they need support. In addition it is a way of monitoring the need for further education and training. The BACP (1999) code of ethics and practice for those using counselling skills in their work clearly recommends that practitioners should be appropriately and sufficiently trained for the counselling skills work they undertake. Training in self-awareness also encourages them to be open to learning from the experience of others and to receive constructive feedback on their own work in such arenas as clinical supervision. The development of interpersonal and intrapersonal awareness is addressed in more detail in Chapter 7, but here I describe the nature of clinical supervision within nursing and the helping professions.

Clinical supervision

Supervision is an established part of practice within many helping disciplines and is indeed part of an already established norm for counsellors, who are continuously supervised throughout their working life. The British Association for Counselling and Psychotherapy (BACP 1998) identifies ongoing supervision as an essential aspect of practice and a requirement for all its members. Recent developments in nursing mean that nursing practice has also been assigned the task of implementing clinical supervision and evidence-based practice (UKCC 1996). It was in 1994 that the Chief Nursing Officer (CNO) for England and Wales endorsed the concept of clinical supervision for nurses, and trust nurse executives were encouraged to implement it throughout their organizations. Following the case of Beverly Allitt, an enrolled nurse who was convicted in 1993/1994 of murdering four babies and other crimes committed in the course of her work, clinical supervision and the monitoring of practice has become a topic of serious debate within the nursing press (Naish 1997). The Clothier report (1994) has also done much to highlight the necessity for adequate standards of supervision, training and education (Rolfe *et al.* 2001).

In 1996 the United Kingdom Central Council for Nursing, Midwifery and Health Visiting (UKCC) issued a position statement on clinical supervision, which made recommendations about its implementation across nursing practice. Linking clinical supervision to the notion of lifelong learning the UKCC (1996) statement was an attempt to formalize what had sometimes been taking place informally. It was a long overdue recognition that people in caring roles need support and caring themselves. As Bishop notes, 'Caring, whether it involves technical skill or personal care, is physically and emotionally wearing and practitioners need sustaining and time for reflection' (2001: 88).

While it is a fairly novel undertaking in nursing, with some specialist areas being more advanced than others, there is evidence to suggest that clinical supervision is now well-established in some practice areas (Butterworth *et al.* 1998; Bishop and Freshwater 2000). Various attempts have been made to describe and define clinical supervision, each highlighting specific aspects of it. In the context of counselling and psychotherapy supervision refers to:

> The opportunity for the counsellor or therapist to discuss his or her work with a more experienced colleague . . . it is not the equivalent of line management . . . supervision should therefore provide an opportunity for a counsellor or therapist to talk about patient or client work without any anxiety that she or he will reprimanded for not working well enough.
>
> (Jacobs 1996: 1)

Bishop's definition contains elements of the purpose of clinical supervision as indicated in the UKCC (1996) position statement. The emphasis is on standards, quality of care, patient safety and protection and staff support. She states it is:

A designated interaction between two or more practitioners, within a safe supportive environment which enables a continuum of reflective, critical analysis of care, to ensure quality patient services.

(Bishop 1998: 8)

Other writers accent the value of supportive clinical supervision in facilitating the lifelong learning of the practitioner. Bond and Holland (1998: 77), for example, say that:

Clinical supervision is a regular, protected time for facilitated, in depth reflection on clinical practice. It aims to enable the supervisee to achieve, sustain and creatively develop a high quality of practice through the means of focused support and development.

Here Bond and Holland (1998) stress the aims of clinical supervision, alluding to its functions. The most often quoted work in relation to the functions of clinical supervision in nursing is that of Proctor's (1986), which identifies three main elements of supervision:

- formative – linked to the process of developing and enhancing skills;
- restorative – linked to the supportive role of supervision;
- normative – linked to the maintenance and improvement of standards.

In essence clinical supervision is widely agreed to be a process through which nurses can reflect on and review their practice, develop and enhance skills and knowledge, while maintaining and improving standards of care (Johns and Freshwater 1998). King observes that supervision offers 'constructive ways of thinking about problems and above all is a safe, confidential place to discuss the work'. Importantly she goes on to say that 'It also offers help in recognising and managing the emotional impact of such work' (1999: 79).

Freshwater (2000a) defines the purpose of clinical supervision as being to:

- provide support for staff members;
- safeguard standards;
- develop professional expertise;
- ensure delivery of quality care.

It also offers an opportunity for the exploration of role conflict by presenting opportunities for reflection on practice, by confirming and validating appropriate practice, by providing a safe environment to express and discuss boundary concerns, and by exploring strategies for role expansion.

Rolfe *et al.* (2001) clarify the difference between models of clinical supervision and modes of practising supervision. Referring to the theoretical and philosophical framework that underpins the approach to supervision they note that models of supervision fall into four main schools of thought derived from the same theories of psychological thought as counselling and psychotherapy. These are psychodynamic, humanistic, cognitive–behavioural and systemic. There is a plethora of literature (within both counselling and nursing) that outlines the models and approaches to clinical supervision; for further information the reader is encouraged to pursue such authors as Bond and Holland (1998), Jacobs (1996) and Holloway (1995).

The modes of supervision, that is the way in which they are implemented, vary in their effectiveness, benefits and limitations. One to one, group, peer and managerial supervision all have their strengths and limitations, many of which are discussed by Rolfe *et al.* (2001; see also Bond and Holland 1998). Whatever the choice of model and mode, a common factor to both counselling and clinical supervision is that of accurate listening. The clinical supervisor therefore also needs to possess the skills of basic counselling in order to facilitate an environment conducive to the safe exploration of clinical practice.

Summary

It is important that nurses familiarize themselves with relevant legal and professional responsibilities before engaging the patient in a counselling relationship. However, it is important for there to be a balance between holding professional knowledge and responding empathically to the patient. For the practitioner to be effective in the use of counselling skills there needs to be a safe, trusting environment, one which is built upon secure foundations. Clearly outlining the boundaries as indicated in this chapter is one way of facilitating an environment within which both the practitioner and the patient can begin to explore the needs of the whole person. Nurses, like other health professionals, are extremely influential in the lives of their patients. Because of this it is legitimate to ask nurses to become more self-aware, as part of their responsibility in the privileged position that practitioners hold.

Not surprisingly then, the last word in this book can rightly be addressed to the needs of the carer. Caring for oneself is a significant concern for all professionals engaged in healthcare, never more so than in the current climate of burnout and workaholism. The RCN working party (1978) noted that nurses in training needed access to a counsellor and that staff counselling was in the main curative rather than preventative. Chapter 7 therefore addresses the implications of nurses developing closer counselling relationships with their patients, together with the personal cost that is sometimes involved.

Chapter **7**

Caring for the carer

It is only relatively recently that certain constraints on the nurse–patient relationship have been relaxed. As late as the 1980s patients were viewed essentially as a biological body to be observed by the nurse, with practitioners being encouraged to maintain an emotional distance from their patients. Traditional approaches to organizing nursing, such as task allocation, were seen as advantageous in that they afforded the nurse some protection from anxiety. Splitting up the daily routine into tasks to be completed reduced the contact and involvement that practitioners had with patients (Menzies-Lyth 1970; Salvage 1995; Briant and Freshwater 1998). Menzies-Lyth (1970) argues that this also served the purpose of desexualizing the nurse–patient relationship, despite the necessity for physical intimacy. As described in Chapter 3 the work of Isobel Menzies-Lyth represented a turning point in understanding nurse–patient interaction. This chapter, building on concepts raised in earlier chapters, draws upon the work of Menzies-Lyth and other nursing theorists in order to address the notion of nursing intimacy. In examining the emotional labour of caring, I also aim to raise awareness of the impact of contemporary policy changes and professional developments on the nurse–patient relationship.

This chapter also attends to the question of what the practitioner does when they need to talk to someone, or when they experience the need for counselling themselves. Exploring the support mechanisms available for practitioners both within and external to their organization I refer to the influence of the organizational culture on nurse–patient interaction. The organizational context and culture is highly significant in any discussion about staff support and development. Menzies-Lyth (1970) suggested that the stressors inherent within nursing were compounded by the organizational ethos, which she argued, worked persistently against the development of a meaningful nurse–patient interaction. Focusing on staff support and development then this chapter examines the interface between the individual practitioner and the collective context, that is the organizational structures within which nursing functions.

Once again a pivotal point in the argument is the concept of self-awareness, and its potential to enable the practitioner to cope with the interpersonal and emotional nature of their often difficult work. Models of reflective practice are identified as one way of supporting the nurse not only in the development of their counselling skills but also in their understanding of interpersonal communications and intrapersonal awareness. 'Intrapersonal' refers to the 'dialogue' that takes place at conscious and unconscious levels within each person, as different aspects of the person express needs and concerns. Such intrapersonal awareness coupled with communication skills may enable the practitioner to seek appropriate support, accept the need for restoration and identify training issues, in order that they may undertake their role with confidence and congruence.

The nurse–patient interaction

When examining the nurse–patient relationship in any great detail the work of Menzies-Lyth (1970, 1988) provides a useful starting point. Three decades ago Menzies-Lyth embarked upon an in-depth research project that exposed some of the systems that nurses had constructed, in order to try and block out of their thinking the psychological difficulties associated with their work (Briant and Freshwater 1998). Based in a London teaching hospital she found a high level of distress, tension and anxiety among nurses, manifest in high attrition rates, high sickness rates and high numbers of students withdrawing from training.

It is interesting to note that recruitment and retention of nurses remains a serious concern today, with many nurses becoming disenchanted with their chosen career for a variety of reasons. Menzies-Lyth (1970: 5) concluded that nursing, by its very nature, was inherently stressful, stating:

> Nurses are in constant contact with people who are physically ill or injured, often seriously. The recovery of patients is not certain and will not always be complete. Nursing patients who have incurable diseases is one of the nurse's most distressing tasks. Nurses are confronted with the threat and the reality of suffering and death, as few lay people are.

She was clear that the techniques practitioners used to contain and modify anxiety were also part of the problem. These included splitting up the nurse–patient relationship and depersonalization of the individual. In order to address this and other problems the modernization of nursing began. In the early 1980s the nursing process, a systematic problem-solving approach to nursing, was introduced. The problem-solving approach was based on individualized care and aimed to facilitate the development of a constructive caring relationship (for an overview of this approach see Arets and Morle 1999).

While clinicians focused their energies on implementing the nursing process, theorists such as Meutzel (1988), Pearson (1988) and McMahon (1991) were developing the notion of a nurse–patient relationship that is founded on mutuality, reciprocity and partnership, including the use of appropriate self-disclosure. This commitment was later reinforced with the implementation of new nursing, which Salvage says: 'explicitly aims to transform interaction between nurses and patients and to promote patients' participation in care'. She goes on to say that the underlying philosophy of new nursing is a 'belief that the relationship between nurse and patient has the potential to be therapeutic and central to the process of recovery' (1995: 9).

Primary nursing is one example of new nursing and, among other things, is based on direct person-to-person communication, with one nurse working with a patient continuously throughout their therapeutic journey. This reduces the number of patients a nurse cares for, and maximizes the amount of time spent with each individual. Primary nursing is a highly complex development and has been contentious, but as Wright contends, it holds the potential for nurses to be able to act therapeutically. The key word here is 'potential', for as Wright cautions, systems of primary nursing are no guarantee in themselves that nursing will be therapeutic. As he rather pointedly argues:

> Having the right system of care in place also seems to require the development of 'right relationships' between employees and their organization, amongst the multidisciplinary team members, within nursing teams and, last but not least, for the nurse to be in right relationship with the self.
>
> (1998: 121)

This movement towards a patient-centred approach to nursing means that the focus of much nursing work has become that of advocacy, and rather than engaging in direct intervention, nurses are encouraged to work with their patients in an empowering partnership. Patient-centred nursing has much in common with Rogers's ([1961]1991) notion of client-centred counselling. Some of these commonalties will become obvious in the subsequent discussion. In patient-centred nursing both nurse and patient, rather than being objectified, are humanized through the co-creation of a mutual alliance.

Patient-centred nursing

In Chapter 3 I referred to the work of Martin Buber (1958) and his exposition of the I–it and I–thou approaches to relationships. It is perhaps pertinent to return to Buber at this point, specifically to illuminate the differences between new nursing and that which was founded upon task allocation. It could be said that nursing that is task-oriented regards the patient as an 'it'. As Kirby and Slevin (1999: 65) put it:

> We are being objective and the person is an object apart from us. We are seeing a set or sum of connected parts. We

are *regarding* an *It*, or a *He* or *She*, but we are not *relating* in any true sense.

(authors' own italics)

In the person-to-person communication inherent within the I–thou stance we are in true relation. Or as Buber terms it, we 'body out' to the other, seeing the other person as a whole. The I–thou way of relating requires that the practitioner is present to the other, that is being with the patient in the moment with spontaneity and immediacy. Acting without a priori knowledge is particularly difficult, because although each patient is a unique individual and as such requires care that is local and contingent, much nursing care is based on standardized protocols and guidelines which, it is assumed, are generalizable. The skill of managing the I–thou nurse–patient relationship is to maintain an awareness of generalizable principles, while being mindful of the unique self–other relationship that is being formed.

However this is more complex than at first it might seem, for as has already been outlined (see Chapter 2), empathic relationships require the nurse to be both involved with the patient and to maintain a type of objectivity. Such objectivity enables the practitioner to provide an appraisal of the patient's situation and offer alternative perspectives. It would seem then that the most effective nurse–patient encounter is one that responds to the patient's whole self but is also able to move between the parts and the whole. Kirby and Slevin capture this movement succinctly when they write that 'True excellence in the nursing relationship can be viewed as this capacity for movement between *I–Thou* and *I–It*, of coming in to *be* and going out to see, as nursing proceeds with a majestic rhythm' (1999: 66, original emphasis). Thus the patient no longer becomes the 'appendectomy in bed 4', 'the bowel washout in cubicle 1' or 'the overdose waiting to be seen' – a fragmented object made up of personal attributes and clinical properties from which nurses can distance themselves.

Contemporary (patient-centred) approaches to nursing and nursing relationships which utilize the practitioner's (and indeed patient's) therapeutic potential have been described as 'the art of nursing' (Parse 1989; Marks-Maran and Rose 1997). Parse (1989) in particular outlines the essentials for practising the art of nursing, including:

- being available to others;
- valuing of the other as a human presence;
- respect for difference;
- ability to connect with others;
- taking pride in self;
- appreciating the mystery of life;
- recognizing joy in the struggles of life;
- resting.

The wider implications of this person-to-person communication have stimulated some debate, not least around the complexities of managing the nurse's own humanity. Meutzel (1988: 11) captures this complexity noting that:

> 'Being there' is that intangible and paradoxically difficult and very simple essence of the dimension of reciprocity and intimacy. It is simple because it is in the desire for closeness of the philanthropic vocation 'to help people', difficult because a closeness that is mutually beneficial in a therapeutic relationship requires mature confrontation by the nurse ... of the vulnerability of her own humanness.

Some writers have expressed their concern about the removal of the protection afforded by task-oriented care (Bowers 1989; Smith 1992). They argue that new approaches to nursing, which emphasize continuity of care, pose specific personal challenges to practitioners, including clarity around professional and personal boundaries. This worry is often associated with the level of emotional involvement that is demanded of the nurse. Indeed Wright questions the morality of unleashing nurses into this type of relationship if it is not adequately supported by managerial commitment to develop the nurse and the environment in which the nurse works. He challenges: 'If the defensive props of tasks are removed, what is put in their place so that the nurse is not physically and psychologically exhausted by their work?' (1998: 121).

These concerns are largely based on the degree of authenticity and presence that the I–Thou interaction demands. However, it would seem that while many nurses are leaving nursing because of disillusionment, there are as many who have become disenchanted with nursing for much deeper reasons, some of which relate to the lack of opportunity available for meaningful relationships with the patient. That nurses actively continue to seek ways of expressing their caring values is manifest in the increasing number of nurses, midwives and health visitors who are training and practising in complementary therapies.

Personal and professional challenges

As already indicated, achieving authenticity and presence within the nurse–patient relationship brings with it a number of challenges. Nurses are skilled performers and can perfect their ability to hide the distress that results from endless restructuring and overwhelming change. Just as nurses 'cope' with the harsh realities of everyday practice, they also appear skilled at concealing the stress of working within an environment that has precious little resources and increasingly diminishing manpower (Salvage 1995). However, when pushed, many nurses have indicated that they would appreciate the services of a counsellor, and in reality where these services are provided many nurses use them (Richelieu 2001).

One problem that faces practitioners is the legitimacy of *their own* feelings, when confronted with the (sometimes extreme) difficulties that their patients experience. In this vein Salvage (1995: 111), reporting the findings of her research, provides an example of a primary nurse who

> described a sense of acute, almost permanent grief that she and other nurses felt for patients who were ill, so much so that it became difficult for nurses to accept their own personal troubles or anxieties as legitimate concerns in the face of greater problems experienced by their patients.

This captures part of the struggle that the practitioner experiences in their quest for authenticity and presence. It is perhaps for this reason that many of the nurses in Salvage's research thought that it would be helpful to have a counsellor attached to each area of practice.

The struggle for authenticity

Authenticity was referred to in Chapter 1, where it was outlined as one of the core conditions of the person-centred approach to counselling (Rogers [1961]1991). Definitions of authenticity often appear to be nebulous and ethereal, in contrast to the concept of inauthenticity, which is seen as dehumanizing relationships. Jean-Paul Sartre (1956), a humanistic existentialist, described inauthenticity as 'bad faith'. This can be best understood as not being true to oneself, or not living one's own humanness. In my research (Freshwater 1999) I found that for many nurses, their humanness was something to ashamed of, leading not only to denial of the authentic self but also to practice being based on bad faith. This has considerable implications for nursing, a profession that is deeply dependent upon the concept of an autonomous, responsible and accountable practitioner (UKCC 1992). Not least there is the question of whether or not the practitioner functioning from a position of bad faith can be truly autonomous.

Although practitioners may not always be conscious of the contradictions between their internal and external worlds, they are often aware of them at some deeper level. Where the barriers to a more intimate caring relationship are removed, and training and support enable an emphasis on the development of self-awareness, it is possible that nurses are gradually confronted with the competing and conflicting tensions inherent within their everyday practice (and within themselves). This awareness brings its own tensions, as being true to oneself is never an easy maxim to follow. Nevertheless, as I have indicated frequently, many writers hold authenticity as central to the development of a true caring relationship (Buber 1958; May 1969; Rogers [1961] 1991). Reflective practice is posited as one way of supporting the practitioner to reconcile such tensions and contradictions and is discussed in more detail below.

The challenge of self-awareness

In considering the notion of an encounter with an other, we need to reflect on that part of the self that is in the role of the nurse. The UKCC's (1996) position statement on clinical supervision and the emphasis on lifelong learning means that all practitioners are committed by their code of ethics (UKCC 1992) to developing self-awareness. Nevertheless, it is fair to say that no one can make anyone else learn. Self-awareness is an invitation to expand one's conscious limits and to become aware of one's own frailties and woundings.

The Greek myth of the wounded healer, Chiron, reminds us that we are all mortal and as such are all wounded in our own individual ways. Kearney, a consultant in palliative care medicine, embraces the concept of the wounded healer, stating: 'We and the other are both there as wounded ones, each searching for healing, and in this reaching out and reaching in we become wounded healers to self as we are wounded healers to others' (1996: 151). Particularly important is Kearney's argument that unless we are able to recognize our own woundedness 'we will mistakenly continue to believe that we as caregivers always have the answers to the other people's problems' (1996: 151).

Being present

'Being present' is closely linked to the development of self-awareness; as Buber notes: 'In order to be able to go out to the other you must have the starting place, you must have been, you must be with yourself' (1958: 72). Presence, like authenticity, is not to be confused with a sentimental attitude towards the patient, but rather it 'depends firmly and consistently on how the nurse conceives of human beings' (Freshwater 1999: 32). Presence then is a way of being, rather than a technique that can be applied. Essentially presence is a gift of both time and self, wonderfully articulated by Kleiman who says 'To alleviate aloneness, this is a most expensive gift. To give this gift of time, and presence in the patient's space, a person has to value the outcomes of relating' (2001: 162). Linking presence with the notion of reflection in action, Boykin (1998) suggests that intentional and authentic presence involves a way of listening and communication that gives of oneself. Presence, she argues, requires practice, can grow through reflection in action, and heightens one's awareness of the moral nature of things.

There are a number of challenges that face the practitioner committed to authentic nursing and presence. These include organizational challenges (linked to power dynamics and hierarchical structures), historical challenges (linked to the dominance discourse of the medical model and positivistic science), and political challenges (linked to the emerging policy initiatives and rationing of resources). As already mentioned, many nurses are leaving the profession, frustrated by the barriers to providing good nursing care. Challenges such as staff shortages (alongside other resource issues such as lack of privacy due to cramped conditions) militate against the development of meaningful nurse–patient relationships, in which counselling skills can be practised. Furthermore they perpetuate the task-oriented approach to nursing. On top of all this nurses often feel unsupported in their day-to-day work, which in itself can inhibit the intention to create a more meaningful interaction with their patients through counselling skills.

Support and development

Throughout this book I have reinforced the point that by practising counselling skills in nursing nurses may find that many of their own needs are brought to the surface. Nurses using counselling skills with their patients will make contact with a range of different emotions, some of which will almost inevitably resonate with the nurse, because nurses are human too. As Stewart notes the practitioner's 'own vibrational chords may be set in vibration by the emotion of the other person' (1983: 21). In Chapter 6 I suggested the importance of clinical supervision in supporting the emotional, physical and developmental needs of the individual. There are however a number of other options that nurses might consider in establishing a network that sufficiently meets their own needs.

Reflective practice

Reflective practice, which continues to grow in popularity across a variety of professions, is now firmly embedded within the language of nursing. However, while it is often referred to within curriculum documents, codes of practice and policy initiatives, many clinicians struggle to engage in what Rolfe *et al.* (2001) term 'critical reflection'.

Reflective practice has its own body of literature, which can be pursued by those who wish to develop the brief discussion of it here (Johns and Freshwater 1998; Rolfe *et al.* 2001; Freshwater 2002). No debate surrounding reflective practice can begin without reference to the work of Donald Schön (1983). His work is of particular relevance in that he writes of reflection *on* action and reflection *in* action. These twin aspects can be linked not only to the notion of clinical supervision, but also to that of the internal supervisor (Casement 1985).

Reflection on action can be defined as 'the retrospective contemplation of practice undertaken in order to uncover the knowledge used in a particular situation, by analysing and interpreting the information recalled (Fitzgerald 1994: 67). While Fitzgerald focuses on the knowledge used in practice situations, other writers are concerned with the development of self through reflection (Freshwater 2000, 2002; Boyd and Fales 1983). Reflection in action involves a much more sophisticated and complex activity; as Rolfe *et al.* point out: 'the advanced practitioner is not only conscious of what she is doing, but also of how she is doing it' (2001: 128). Just as empathy can be separated into basic and advanced empathy, reflection can also be divided (albeit artificially) into basic reflection on action and deeper reflection in action. Reflection on and in action both facilitate the emergence of the internal supervisor, which can be used in practice to watch, listen and understand ourselves, as well our patients.

I have noted elsewhere that 'reflective practice provides a way for caring individuals to explore and confront their own caring beliefs and how these are executed in practice'. Moreover 'it is about transforming self and thereby caring in practice' (Freshwater 1999: 29). The fact that reflective practice involves a transformation of self means that it may represent a threat to many practitioners, who largely survive understandably by the defence of not allowing themselves to reflect too deeply about their own responses to patients (Burridge 1996). Burridge links such defensiveness to institutionalized attitudes towards not coping, which is deemed by such organizations to be negative.

While it is not surprising that reflective practice brings about a degree of fear in practitioners, this makes it difficult when it comes to supervision, because for many authors reflective practice is pivotal to the success of clinical supervision (Binnie and Titchen 1995; Johns and Freshwater 1998; Fitzgerald 2000; Rolfe *et al.* 2001). Currently both clinical supervision and reflective practice are viewed with suspicion and cynicism within nursing. Where the uptake of supervision is high, practitioners often face conflict and sabotage from their colleagues (Freshwater *et al.* 2001). Whereas ongoing supervision is a requirement for practising counsellors, it is as yet only a recommendation for nurses and health visitors. Although midwives have been involved in supervision for a number of years, many would agree that this is mainly managerial supervision, as opposed to a regular protected time for reflection on practice. It is true that not every nurse uses counselling skills in their everyday practice; as such supervision remains an option for those practitioners who choose to extend their role to include the skills of counselling. However, Bond and Holland draw parallels between clinical supervision in counselling and nursing. They argue that 'nursing is essentially about relationships, with both clients and colleagues, and there are similar needs for practitioners to develop self-awareness and interpersonal and emotional skills to cope with the often stressful nature of their work' (1998: 25). Clinical supervision is potentially of benefit to all the tasks involved in nursing.

Training and education

One of the functions of reflective practice and clinical supervision is that of enabling the practitioner to identify their own professional development needs and translate these into action. This includes the identification of further training and education. Nurses wishing to learn counselling skills to complement their practice can embark upon training programmes to help them get started, and those practitioners already using counselling skills may find that they wish to refine and fine-tune their skills, or develop specialist counselling skills (such as bereavement counselling). The courses available are numerous and vary in length, focus and quality, while many nurses will be encouraged to take courses provided by the local workforce confederation; it is worth exploring what else is on offer (see the information section at the end of this book).

Counselling

Many nurses have embarked upon professional training to become counsellors and have experienced personal therapy as part of that training. Personal counselling is a basic requirement for any counsellor wishing to become accredited. Nurses, however, do not have any such requirement; registration instead is based on the achievement of competencies identified by professional regulating bodies. Where a practitioner identifies a need for counselling it is important to that appropriate resources and information are at hand. Many NHS settings now provide some kind of staff counselling service, and for those who would rather seek support from an external source there are many organizations, which can provide lists of registered and accredited counsellors (see the addresses in the Appendix).

Other forms of support

Following the successful introduction of their nursing development unit, Purdy *et al.* (1988) identified ways of creating support mechanisms for nurses engaged in therapeutic nursing. While these do not specifically have the use of counselling skills in mind, they can be seen to be relevant to the support and development of the practitioner, either who is interested in using counselling skills within their practice or who is seeking additional emotional and psychological sustenance. They include the formation of on-site peer groups, support teams to provide counselling, the setting up of extensive staff development, and applying maximum resources to improving the working environment.

At times of distress practitioners often turn to their colleagues for support. This can be seen in critical incident debriefing following such traumas as a cardiac arrest. It usually occurs on an ad hoc basis, with nurses seeking out those colleagues with whom they feel safe and supported. In some cases staff support groups are organized, although currently little is known about the value of such groups. Burridge, commenting on the role of staff support groups in psychiatry, observes that 'in the same way that staff rarely reveal their vulnerable self in a staff support group, nor do they share their feelings of anger, jealousy, envy etc.' He goes on to report:

> I have sat through week after week of staff groups where an hour and a quarter has been spent complaining bitterly about the hospital managers. At no point did anyone manage to ask us what we were avoiding or indeed point out that we were avoiding anything.
>
> (1996: 387)

Challenging institutional attitudes demands a great deal of commitment and energy and support from peers and colleagues. Confronting the organizational and professional culture of coping, and avoiding the pressure to work additional hours, are some ways of evading burnout. It is said that we teach what we most need to learn; as nurses it is important that we provide a role model to our patients of ways of being healthy. Thus the practitioner is urged to attend to their physical, psychological, emotional and spiritual needs in order that they may live themselves in the way in which they would wish their patients to live. If it did not sound too moralistic I would be tempted to write that we must practise what we preach!

Summary

There is little doubt about the benefit of creating an environment in which the nurse–patient relationship is given the attention it deserves. The use of counselling skills in nursing may not only benefit the patient, but also enable the nurse to deepen the significance of and find meaning in their everyday practice. Further, the nurse engaged in such activities has the opportunity to expand and learn more about themselves as human beings. As Stewart (1983: 22) comments:

Nursing as a profession must surely benefit if the nurse is recognised as a person who counsels as part of her clinical role. If there is a benefit to the individual nurse there will be a cumulative benefit brought about through increased awareness and understanding of how patient needs are related to her own.

There are significant differences between working with someone as a client in formal counselling and the appropriate use of counselling skills within one's primary role. The main differences lie in setting boundaries, being clear about the focus of the relationship and the professional's role within it, and knowing the limitations of the time and skills that are on offer. This book has shown that all these aspects have some part to play in nursing, even if they are not so formally spelt out. Both the practice of counselling, and the role of the nurse using counselling skills are rewarding, though sometimes taxing. This is why the provision of counselling skills carries with it implications for training, education and professional support, which need to be taken as seriously as the use of the skills themselves.

For a nurse to make effective use of counselling skills they need to be able to create a trusting environment in which the patient can feel safe enough to explore their concerns. The skills outlined in this book, when used appropriately and in context, can help the practitioner to create that environment. In addition to the education and training in counselling skills that nurses might undertake, they also require systematic support through clinical supervision, and the provision of relevant support services.

Appendix

Useful information

Albany Trust Counselling
280 Balham High Street
London
SW17 7AL

Provides counselling for sexual identity problems.

Alcoholics Anonymous
PO Box 1
Stonebow House
Stonebow
York
YO1 2NJ

Telephone: 01904 644026 (UK)
Website: www.alcoholics-anonymous.org.uk

British Association for Counselling and Psychotherapy
1 Regent Place
Rugby
Warwickshire
CV21 2VT

Telephone: 0870 4435252
Fax: 0870 4435160
E-mail: bacp@bacp.co.uk
Website: www.bacp.co.uk

Brooks Advisory Centres
165 Grays Inn Road
London
WC1X 8UD

Telephone: 0207 713 9000
Helpline: 0207 617 8000
Website: www.brookcentres.org.uk

Provides information and counselling about sexual problems, contraception and pregnancy.

Cancer BACUP
3 Bath Place
Rivington Street
London
EC2A 3DR

Website: www.bacup.org.uk

Childline
Headquarters
Studd Street
London
N1 0QW

Website: www.childline.org.uk

Cruse Bereavement Care
Cruse House
126 Sheen Road
Richmond
Surrey
TW9 1UR

Provides bereavement counselling

Department of Health
Information Division
5th Floor
Skipton House
80 London Road
Elephant and Castle
London
SE1 6LW

Disabledinfo.com
60 Ebury Street
London
SW1
Website: www.disabledinfo.com

Faculty of Healthcare Counsellors and Psychotherapists
Telephone: 0870 4435252
Email: fhcp@bacp.co.uk

Health Online
The Chambers
Threfalls Building
Trueman Street
Liverpool
L3 2BA
Website: www.health-online.uk.com

Haven Trust

Telephone: 020 7384 0000
National Helpline: 08707 272273
Website: thehaventrust.org.uk

Provides support to people affected by breast cancer.

Health Promotion England
50 Eastbourne Terrace
London
W2 3QR
Website: www.hpe.org.uk

MIND
Granta House
15–19 Broadway
London
E15 4BQ

Telephone: 0208 522 1728
Helpline: 0345 660163
Website: www.mind.org.uk

National AIDS Trust
New City Cloisters
198 Old Street
London
EC1V 9FR
Website: nat.org.uk

National Healing UK Ltd.
PO Box 3718
Colchester
Essex
CO3 5UB

Website: www.healthypages.co.uk

Nurseline

Telephone: 020 7647 3463
Email: nurseline@rcn.org.uk

Provides independent advice and support for nurses and midwives.

Nursing and Midwifery Council
23 Portland Place
London
W1B 1PZ
Telephone: 020 763 7181
Fax: 020 7436 2924

Website: www.nmc-uk.org

Replacing the United Kingdom Central Council for Nursing, Midwifery and Health Visiting.

Royal College of Nursing Counselling Service
Telephone: 0845 7697064

Provides free confidential counselling for nurses.

Samaritans
10 The Grove
Slough
SL1 1QP
Telephone: 01753 532713
Helpline: 0345 909090 (UK)
Website: www.samaritans.org

Terrence Higgins Trust
52–54 Grays Inn Road
London
WC1X 8JE

Website: www.tht.org.uk

UK Self help directory
Website: www.ukselfhelp.info

WING (Work Injured Nurses Group)
Telephone: 0207 647 3465
Email: WING@rcn.org.uk

Provides support and advice for nurses who have illness or injury as a result of work.

References

Arets, A. and Morle, K. (1999) The nursing process: an introduction, in L. Basford and O. Slevin (eds) *Theory and Practice of Nursing*. Cheltenham: Stanley Thornes.

Beauchamp, T.L. and Childress, J.F. (1983) *Principles of Biomedical Ethics*. Oxford: Oxford University Press.

Beck, A.T. (1976) *Cognitive Therapy and Emotional Disorders*. New York: International Universities Press.

Benner, P. (1984) *From Novice to Expert*. Menlo Park, CA: Addison Wesley.

Binnie, A. and Titchen, A. (1995) The art of clinical supervision, *British Journal of Nursing*, 4: 327–34.

Bishop, V. (1998) Clinical supervision: what is it? in V. Bishop (ed.) *Clinical Supervision in Practice*. London: Palgrave.

Bishop, V. (2001) Professional development and clinical supervision, in V. Bishop and I. Scott (eds) *Challenges in Clinical Practice*. Basingstoke: Palgrave.

Bishop, V. and Freshwater, D. (2000) *Clinical Supervision: Examples and Pointers for Good Practice*. Report for Leicester Hospitals Education Consortium. Leicester: Mary Seacole Research Centre, De Monfort University.

Bohm, D. (1990) *On Dialogue*. London: Routledge.

Bond, M. and Holland, S. (1998) *Skills of Clinical Supervision for Nurses*. Buckingham: Open University Press.

Bowers, L. (1989) The significance of primary nursing, *Journal of Advanced Nursing*, 14: 13–19.

Bowman, G.S. and Thompson, D. (1998) Therapeutic nursing in acute care, in R. McMahon and A. Pearson (eds) *Nursing as Therapy*. Cheltenham: Stanley Thornes.

Boyd, E. and Fales, A. (1983) Reflective learning: the key to learning from experience, *Journal of Humanistic Psychology*, 23 (2): 99–117.

Boykin, A. (1998) Nursing as caring through the reflective lens, in C. Johns and D. Freshwater (eds) *Transforming Nursing through Reflective Practice*. Oxford: Blackwell Science.

Briant, S. and Freshwater, D. (1998) Exploring mutuality in the nurse–patient relationship, *British Journal of Nursing*, 7 (4): 204–11.

British Association for Counselling and Psychotherapy (BACP) (1998) *Code of ethics and practice for counsellors*. Rugby: BACP.

British Association for Counselling and Psychotherapy (BACP) (1999) *Code of ethics and practice for those using counselling skills in their work*. Rugby: BACP.

Buber, M. (1958) *I and Thou*, 2nd edn. Edinburgh: T. and T. Clark.

Bucknall, A. (2001) Integrating psychological therapies in primary care, *HealthCare Counselling and Psychotherapy Journal*, 1 (1): 27–9.

Burnard, P. (1990) *Learning Human Skills. An Experiential Guide for Nurses*, 2nd edn. Oxford: Butterworth Heinemann.

Burnard, P. (1992) *Counselling: A Guide to Practice in Nursing*. Oxford: Butterworth Heinemann.

Burnard, P. (1995) Counselling, or being a counsellor? *Professional Nurse*, January: 261–2.

Burnard, P. (1998a) Listening as a personal quality, *Journal of Community Nursing*, 12 (2): 32–4.

Burnard, P. (1998b) Personal qualities or skills? A report of a study of nursing students' views of the characteristics of counsellors, *Nurse Education Today*, 18: 649–54.

Burridge, T. (1996) Through a glass darkly: some reflections on psychiatric nursing, *Psychodynamic Counselling*, 2 (3): 376–90.

Butterworth, T., White, E., Carson, J., Jeacock, J. and Clements, A. (1998) Developing and evaluating clinical supervision in the United Kingdom, *EDTNA/ERCA Journal*, 24 (1): 208.

Carkhuff, R.R. (1987) *The Art of Helping*, 6th edn. Amherst: Human Resource Development Press.

Carlssoin, R., Lindberg, G., Westin, L. and Israelsson, B. (1997) Influence of coronary nursing management follow up on lifestyle after acute myocardial infarction, *Heart*, 77: 256–59.

Casement, P. (1985) *On Learning from the Patient*. London: Routledge.

Childs-Clarke, A. (1994) Nursing care of bulimia with cognitive behavioural therapy, *Nursing Times*, 90 (40): 40–2.

Clothier, C., MacDonald, C.A. and Shaw, D.A. (1994) *The Allitt Inquiry*. London: HMSO.

Cole, S. (2001) A place for person centred therapy, *HealthCare Counselling and Psychotherapy Journal*, 1 (1): 11–13.

Cook, P. (2001) Children, and their families, in intensive care, *HealthCare Counselling and Psychotherapy Journal*, 1 (1): 14–17.

Department of Health (DoH) (1998) *A First Class Service: Quality in the New NHS*. Wetherby: DoH.

Department of Health (1999) *The National Service Framework for Mental Health*. London: DoH.

Department of Health (DoH) (2000) *The NHS Plan: A Plan for Investment. A Plan for Reform*. Norwich: The Stationery Office.

Dilworth, S. (2000) Boundaries not barriers: having the confidence to confide in clinical supervision, in D. Freshwater (ed.) *Making a Difference*. Portsmouth: Nursing Praxis International.

Egan, G. (1994) The Skilled Helper, *A Problem Management Approach to Helping*, 5th edn. Belmont, CA: Brooks/Cole.

Ellis, A. (1990) *Reason and Emotion in Psychotherapy*. New York: Citadel Press.

Ewles, L. and Simnett, I. (1995) *Promoting Health*, 3rd edn. London: Scutari Press.

Festinger, L. (1957) *A Theory of Cognitive Dissonance*. New York: Harper and Row.

Fitzgerald, M. (1994) Theories of reflection for learning, in A. Palmer, S. Burns and C. Bulman (eds) *Reflective Practice in Nursing*. Oxford: Blackwell Science.

Fitzgerald, M. (2000) Clinical supervision and reflective practice, in C. Bulman and S. Burns (eds) *Reflective Practice in Nursing*, 2nd edn. Oxford: Blackwell Science.

French, P. (1983) *Social Skills for Nursing Practice*. Kent: Croom Helm.

Freshwater, D. (1998) From acorn to oak tree: a neoplatonic perspective of reflection, *Australian Journal of Holistic Nursing*, 5 (2): 14–19.

Freshwater, D. (1999) Communicating with self through caring: the student nurse's experience of reflective practice, *International Journal of Human Caring*, 3 (3): 28–33.

Freshwater, D. (2000) *Transformatory Learning in Nurse Education*. Portsmouth: Nursing Praxis International.

Freshwater, D. (2002) *Therapeutic Nursing. Improving Patient Care through Reflective Practice*. London: Sage.

Freshwater, D. and Rolfe, G. (2001) Critical reflexivity: a politically and ethically engaged research method for nursing, *NTResearch*, 6 (1): 526–37.

Freshwater, D., Storey, L. and Walsh, L. (2001) *Establishing Clinical Supervision in Prison Healthcare*. Report for the Prison Policy Taskforce, Foundation of Nursing Studies and UKCC.

Freud, S. (1915) *The Unconscious*, Standard Edition, 12: 159–204.

Freud, S. (1923) *The Ego and the Id*, Penguin Freud Library, Vol. 11. Harmondsworth: Penguin.

Freud, S. ([1933]1964) *New Introductory Lectures on Psychoanalysis*, Standard Edition, 22. London: Hogarth.

Gaston, M. (2001a) The psychological impact of a heart attack, *Faculty of Healthcare Counsellors and Psychotherapy Journal*, Spring. Rugby: BACP.

Gaston, M. (2001b) Counselling – a crucial part of cardiac rehabilitation, *HealthCare Counselling and Psychotherapy Journal*, 1 (1): 43–4.

Gordon, P. (1999) *Face to Face. Therapy as Ethics*. London: Constable.

Great Britain Parliament (1972) *Report of a Committee on Nursing*. Chairman Professor Asa Briggs. London: HMSO.

Guggenbahl-Craig, A. (1978) *Power in the Helping Professions*. Dallas, TX: Spring.

Hargie, O., Saunders, C. and Dickson, D. (1986) *Social Skills in Interpersonal Communication*. London: Croom Helm.

Heath, H. and Freshwater, D. (2000) Clinical supervision as an emancipatory process: avoiding inappropriate intent, *Journal of Advanced Nursing*, 35 (5): 1298–306.

Henderson, V.A. (1966) *The Nature of Nursing*. New York: National League for Nursing Press.

Heron, J. (1989) *The Facilitator's Handbook*. London: Kogan Page.

Holloway, E. (1995) *Clinical Supervision: A Systems Approach*. London: Sage.

Horder, J. and Moore, G.T. (1990) The consultation and outcome, *British Journal of General Practice*, 40: 442–3.

Hough, M. (1994) *A Practical Approach to Counselling*. London: Pitman.

Jacobs, M. (1991) *Psychodynamic Counselling in Action*. London: Sage.

Jacobs, M. (ed.) (1996) *In Search of Supervision*. Buckingham: Open University Press.

Jacobs, M. (1999) *Swift to Hear*, 2nd edn. London: SPCK.

Jacoby, M. (1984) *The Analytic Encounter. Transference and Human Relationship*. Toronto: Inner City Books.

Johns, C. (1998) Opening the doors of perception, in C. Johns and D. Freshwater (eds) *Transforming Nursing through Reflective Practice*. Oxford: Blackwell Science.

Johns, C. and Freshwater, D. (1998) *Transforming Nursing through Reflective Practice*. Oxford: Blackwell Science.

Jones, A. (1970) *School Counselling in Practice*. London: Ward Lock International.

Jones, A. (1993) A first step in effective communication: providing a supportive environment for counselling in hospital, *Professional Nurse*, 8 (8): 501–5.

Jones, L. and Cribb, A. (1997) Ethical issues in health promotion, in J. Katz and A. Peberdy (eds) *Promoting Health: Knowledge and Practice*. Basingstoke: Macmillan.

Jourard, S.M. (1971) *The Transparent Self*. Princeton, NJ: Nostrand.

Kearney, M. (1996) *Mortally Wounded*. New York: Touchstone.

Kelly, G.A. (1995) *The Psychology of Personal Constructs*. New York: Norton.

King, G. (1999) *Counselling Skills for Teachers*. Buckingham: Open University Press.

Kirby, C. (1999) The therapeutic relationship, in L. Basford and O. Slevin (eds) *Theory and Practice of Nursing*. Cheltenham: Stanley Thornes.

Kirby, C. and Slevin, O. (1999) Commitment to care, in Basford, L. and Slevin, O. (eds) *Theory and Practice of Nursing. An Integrated Approach to Nursing Care*. Cheltenham: Stanley Thornes.

Kleiman, S. (2001) Josephine Paterson and Loretta Zderad. Humanistic nursing theory with clinical applications, in M. Parker (ed.) *Nursing Theories and Nursing Practice*. Philadelphia, PA: F.A. Davis.

Landsdown, R. (1996) *Children in Hospital.* Oxford: Oxford University Press.

McLeod, J. (1993) *An Introduction to Counselling.* Buckinghamshire: Open University Press.

Macleod Clark, J., Kendall, S. and Haverty, S. (1992) Effective use of health education skills, in E. Horne and T. Cowen (eds) *Effective Communication: Some Nursing Perspectives.* London: Wolfe.

McMahon, R. (1991) Therapeutic nursing: theories, issues and practice, in R. McMahon and A. Pearson (eds) *Nursing as Therapy.* London: Chapman and Hall.

McMahon, R. and Pearson, A. (eds) (1998) *Nursing as Therapy,* 2nd edn. Cheltenham: Stanley Thornes.

Mager, R.F. (1962) *Preparing Instructional Objectives.* Palo Alto, CA: Fearon.

Marks-Maran, D. and Rose, P. (1997) *Reconstructing Nursing. Beyond Art and Science.* London: Balliere Tindall.

Maslow, A. (1968) *Towards a Psychology of Being,* 2nd edn. Toronto: Van Nostrand.

Maslow, A. (1970) *Motivation and Personality,* 2nd edn. New York: Harper and Row.

May, R. (1969) *Love and Will.* New York: W.W. Norton.

Menzies-Lyth, I.A.P. (1970) *The Functioning of Social Systems as a Defence against Anxiety.* London: Tavistock Institute.

Menzies-Lyth, I.A.P. (1988) *Containing Anxiety in Institutions.* London: Free Association Books.

Meutzel, P.A. (1988) Therapeutic Nursing, in A. Pearson (ed.) *Primary Nursing in the Burford and Oxford Nursing Development Units.* London: Chapman and Hall.

Naidoo, J. and Wills, J. (1994) *Health Promotion: Foundations for Practice.* London: Balliere Tindall.

Naish, J. (1997) Dangerous assumptions, *Nursing Times,* 93 (46): 37–8.

Nightingale, F. (1859) *Notes on Nursing: What It Is and What It Is Not.* Philadelphia, PA: Lippincott.

Orem, D.E. (1971) *Nursing: Concepts of Practice.* New York: McGraw-Hill.

Orem, D.E. (1990) A nursing practice theory in three parts, 1956–1989, in M. Parker (ed.) *Nursing Theories in Practice.* New York: National League for Nursing Press.

Palmer, R.L., Chaloner, D.A. and Oppenheimer, R. (1992) Childhood sexual experiences with adults reported by female psychiatric patients. *British Journal of Psychiatry,* 160: 261–5.

Palmer, S., Dainbow, S. and Milner, P. (1996) *Counselling: The BAC Counselling Reader.* London: Sage.

Parker, M. (ed.) (2001) *Nursing Theories and Nursing Practice.* Philadelphia, PA: F.A. Davis.

Parse, R.R. (1989) Essentials for practising the art of nursing, *Nursing Science Quarterly,* 2 (3): 111.

Parse, R.R. (1998) *The Human Becoming School of Thought: A Perspective for Nurses and Other Health Professionals.* Thousand Oaks, CA: Sage.

Parse, R.R. (2001) The human becoming school of thought, in M. Parker (ed.) *Nursing Theories and Nursing Practice*. Philadelphia, PA: F.A. Davis.

Parsons, T. (1966) On becoming a patient, in J.R. Folta and E.S. Deck (eds) *A Sociological Framework for Patient Care*. New York: John Wiley and Son.

Paterson, J.G. and Zderad, L.T. (1976) *Humanistic Nursing*. New York: John Wiley.

Paterson, J.G. and Zderad, L.T. (1988) *Humanistic Nursing*, 2nd edn. New York: National League for Nursing Press.

Pearson, A. (1988) Primary nursing, in A. Pearson (ed.) *Primary Nursing in the Burford and Oxford Nursing Development Units*. London: Chapman and Hall.

Peplau, H.E. (1962) Interpersonal techniques: the crux of psychiatric nursing, *American Journal of Nursing*, 62: 50–4.

Peplau, H.E. ([1952]1988) *Interpersonal Relations in Nursing*. London: Macmillan.

Prochaska, J. and DiClemente, C. (1984) *The Transtheoretical Approach: Crossing Traditional Boundaries of Therapy*. New York: Daw Jones Irwin.

Proctor, B. (1986) *Supervision: A Working Alliance*. Sussex: Alexia.

Purdy, J. (1988) Caring for nurses. Unpublished MA thesis, University of Nottingham.

Raleigh, E.H. and Odtohan, B.C. (1987) The effects of cardiac teaching programme on teaching rehabilitation, *Heart and Lung*, 16: 311–17.

Remen, R.N. (1996) *Kitchen Table Wisdom*. London: Pan Books.

Richards, D. and McDonald, B. (1990) *Behavioural Psychotherapy*. Oxford: Heinemann.

Richelieu, M. (2001) Counselling NHS staff, *HealthCare Counselling and Psychotherapy Journal*, 1 (1): 37.

Rogers, C.R. ([1961]1991) *Client Centred Therapy*. London: Constable.

Rolfe, G., Freshwater, D. and Jasper, M. (2001) *Critical Reflection for Nursing and the Helping Professions*. Palgrave: Basingstoke.

Royal College of Nursing (RCN) (1978) *Counselling in Nursing*. London: Royal College of Nursing.

Sartre, J.P. (1956) *Being and Nothingness*. New York: Philosophical Library.

Salvage, J. (1995) *Nursing Intimacy. An Ethnographic Approach to Nurse–Patient Interaction*. London: Scutari Press.

Sayce, E. (1993) Given a voice, *Nursing Times*, 89 (36): 48–50.

Schön, D.A. (1983) *The Reflective Practitioner*. London: Temple Smith.

Seedhouse, D. (1988) *Ethics: The Heart of Health Care*. London: Wiley.

Sidell, M. (1997) Supporting individuals and facilitating change: the role of counselling skills, in J. Katz and A. Peberdy (eds) *Promoting Health*. Buckingham: Open University Press.

Skinner, B.F. (1953) *Science and Human Behaviour*. London: Macmillan.

Slevin, O. (1995) Therapeutic intervention in nursing, in L. Basford and O. Slevin (eds) *Theory and Practice of Nursing*. Cheltenham: Stanley Thornes.

Smith, P. (1992) *The Emotional Labour of Nursing. How Nurses Care.* Basingstoke: Macmillan.

Smith, S. and Norton, K. (1999) *Counselling Skills for Doctors.* Buckingham: Open University Press.

Soohbany, M.S. (1996) Quest for a counselling paradigm in nursing. Unpublished MSc Dissertation, University of Bristol.

Soohbany, M.S. (1999) Counselling as part of nursing fabric: where is the evidence? A phenomenological study using 'reflection on actions' as a tool for framing the 'lived counselling experiences of nurses', *Nurse Education Today*, 19: 35–40.

Stewart, W. (1983) *Counselling in Nursing. A Problem Solving Approach.* London: Harper and Row.

Stockwell, F. (1972) *The Unpopular Patient.* London: Royal College of Nursing.

Thompson, D.R. (1990) *Counselling the Coronary Patient and Partner.* London: Scutari Press.

Trower, P., Casey, A. and Dryden, W. (1990) *Cognitive Behavioural Counselling in Action.* London: Sage.

Tschudin, V. (1996) *Counselling Skills for Nurses*, 4th edn. London: Balliere Tindall

Turney, C., Owens, L.C., Hatton, N., Williams, G. and Cairns, L.G. (1976) *Sydney Micro Skills: Series 2 Handbook.* Sydney: Sydney University Press.

United Kingdom Central Council for Nursing, Midwifery and Health Visiting (UKCC) (1992) *Code of Conduct for the Nurse, Midwife and Health Visitor.* London: UKCC.

United Kingdom Central Council for Nursing, Midwifery and Health Visiting (UKCC) (1996) *Position Statement on Cinical Supervision for Nursing and Health Visiting.* London: UKCC.

Van Ooijen, E. and Charnock, A. (1994) *Sexuality and Patient Care: A Guide for Nurses and Teachers.* London: Chapman and Hall.

Watson, J. (1979) *Nursing: The Philosophy and Science of Caring.* Boston, MA: Little, Brown.

Winnicott, D.W. (1965) *Maturational Processes and the Facilitating Environment.* London: Hogarth Press.

Wright, S. (1998) Facilitating therapeutic nursing and independent practice, in R. McMahon and A. Pearson (eds) *Nursing as Therapy.* Cheltenham: Stanley Thornes.

Zinschitz, E. (1998) The person centred approach in work with disabled persons, *Counselling*, August: 210–16.

Index

AN INTRODUCTION TO COUNSELLING
THIRD EDITION
John McLeod (editor)

Reviews of the second edition:

... It is impossible to do justice to such an exhaustive, broadbased and very readable work in a short review. Professor McLeod has been meticulous, and with true scientific impartiality has looked at, studied and described the many strands and different schools of thought and methods that can lead towards successful counselling

Therapy Weekly

... This is a fascinating, informative, comprehensive and very readable book ... McLeod has produced a text that offers a great deal no matter what your level of competence or knowledge

Journal of Interprofessional Care

... one of the book's strengths is McLeod's willingness to go beyond a history of the development of counselling or a beginner's technical manual ... [and to] consider the political dimensions of counselling and the relevance of power to counselling relationships. A worthwhile acquisition for therapeutic community members, whatever their discipline or background

Therapeutic Communities

This thoroughly revised and expanded version of the bestselling text, *An Introduction to Counselling*, provides a comprehensive introduction to the theory and practice of counselling and therapy. It is written in a clear, accessible style, covers all the core approaches to counselling, and takes a critical, questioning approach to issues of professional practice. Placing each counselling approach in its social and historical context, the book also introduces a wide range of contemporary approaches, including narrative therapy, systemic, feminist and multicultural.

This third edition includes a new chapter on the important emerging approach of philosophical counselling, and a chapter on the counselling relationship, as well as expanded coverage of attachment theory, counselling on the Internet, and solution-focused therapy. The text has been updated throughout, with additional illustrative vignettes and case studies.

Current, comprehensive and readable, *An Introduction to Counselling* is a classic introduction to its subject.

Contents

c.464pp   0 335 21189 5 (Paperback)   0 335 21190 9 (Hardback)

REFLECTIVE PRACTICE
A GUIDE FOR NURSES AND MIDWIVES

Beverley J. Taylor

Reflection helps us understand the impact of our actions and improve our professional skills. This practical guide shows nurses and midwives how to develop a reflective approach to their work and how to sustain reflective practice throughout their professional lives.

Bev Taylor introduces three main types of reflection: technical, practical and emancipatory, showing readers how these can be used in different aspects of clinical work. She acknowledges the issues faced by practitioners in bureaucratic work settings with time constraints and regulated routines, and shows how reflection can help professionals deal with the complexity of their working lives. Readers are given a 'kitbag' of strategies they can use to get started.

With great warmth Bev Taylor describes how developing a reflective practice is part of learning how to value yourself as a nurse or midwife, and as a person. Throughout the book she provides real examples of reflective writing from nurses and midwives, and shows how these professionals have been able to improve their skills as a result of being alert to their practice.

> A practical and insightful guide, richly illuminated with stories from everyday practice, to enable the practitioner to become an effective reflective practitioner. The power of Bev Taylor's approach is to view reflection as a way of life and not just as a technique.
> Christopher Johns, Reader in Advanced Nursing Practice,
> University of Luton, UK

> Bev Taylor's latest work weaves a tapestry for a reflective frame as foundational to our humanity, restoring and integrating the personal with our professional life, work and experiences . . . It is a hopeful framework and a healing gift to all practising nurses and midwives.
> Jean Watson, Distinguished Professor of Nursing,
> University of Colorado, USA

Contents
The nature of reflection – The nature of nursing and midwifery – Getting ready to reflect – Practitioners' reflections on their personal histories – The value of reflection – Types of reflection – Technical reflection – Practical reflection – Emancipatory reflection – Experiences and reflections – Maintaining reflective practice – References – Index.

272pp   0 335 20689 1 (Paperback)   0 335 20690 5 (Hardback)

DEVELOPING COMMUNITY NURSING PRACTICE
Sue Spencer, John Unsworth and Wendy Burke (eds)

Developing Community Nursing Practice is the first book to identify and debate the key issues around community nurses taking responsibility for developing the ways in which they deliver care. Modern health care expects the individual practitioner to develop patient-focused, accessible and evidence-based community services. Despite the fact that the introduction and management of change is now a feature of professional education, community nurses often feel ill-prepared for introducing change in the real world, perceiving a gap between theory and practice. *Developing Community Nursing Practice* aims to close that gap.

This book interweaves thinking about change and innovation with wide-ranging case study experience of contemporary community nursing. It addresses often neglected issues in practice development such as evaluation and sustainability. It gives guidance on how to identify what aspects of practice need to be developed; on how to convince others of the need to change; on how to work across organizational boundaries; and on the likely hazards and how to tackle them.

This is a key resource for all student and practising community nurses (across all specialisms), providing information on how to initiate and implement change and on how ultimately to succeed in developing their own practice.

Contents
Introduction – Part one: Triggering the development of practice – Developing primary care: the influence of society, policy and the professions – Evidence for development – Part two: The process of developing practice – Managing the development of practice – Concepts of risk in the development of practice – Education for change – Part three: Key issues when developing practice – Can you feel the force? The importance of power in the development of practice – It ain't what you do, it's the way that you do it: new and different approaches to practice – References – Index.

224pp   0 335 20557 7 (Paperback)   0 335 20558 5 (Hardback)